Cancer and Energy Medicine: A Healing Journey

Dianne Faure

EEM-AP, LMT, JD

Contents

Part I: Dancing With Death

Part II: Mounting a Defense

This book is dedicated to:
my fellow warriors who have fought and lost their battles,
to those who are fighting on the frontline now,
and to the ones who love them.

Theme Park

I now ride the roller coaster of hope and despair –
the main attraction, frequented by so many,
in this theme park called Cancer.

Admission to this terrible, well-known venue is free –
one stumbles unawares into its penal environs.
The trick then being to find your way out,
not unscathed, but without paying the ultimate fee.

One diligently checks and re-checks the perimeter fence
for a gap, a weakness, a helping hand from the other side.
Clearly a ransom is to be paid in flesh –
one way or another.

I am prepared to climb through a barbed barrier –
not all, but others have done it.
So, why not me?
I too, also, among those called "Survivors."

— Lloyd Howell

Introduction

Have you or someone you love been diagnosed with cancer? Receiving a cancer diagnosis is shocking and overwhelming. No one gives you a roadmap to help you navigate the complicated, tumultuous journey that lies ahead. After the initial shock has worn off, there are batteries of appointments, tests, and procedures before the actual treatment begins. How can you prepare yourself mentally and physically for what lies ahead? How do you know you're making the best decisions about your treatment? What if someone laid down, step by step, what to expect as you travel the scary, dreary road of chemo, surgery, radiation, and recovery? What if there were simple things you or your loved ones could do that could help that journey become less painful, less treacherous, and possibly, less fatal? If you want some insight into these questions, then this book is for you!

While no two people or cancers are the same, *Cancer and Energy Medicine: A Healing Journey* can serve as a roadmap to help you answer frequent questions that crop up during cancer treatment such as:

- How can I prepare my body for the tests, procedures, and infusions I will encounter?
- What will chemotherapy feel like?
- How will my body change over time?
- What side effects can I expect?
- Are there ways to manage those side effects without medication?
- How do I advocate for myself in difficult circumstances?
- What alternative modalities could help me manage my cancer treatment and the side effects that come with it?
- How painful might surgery be and how long does it take to heal?

- What can I expect from radiation?

- What types of late effects are common post-treatment?

- Are there strategies to help prevent me from falling victim to permanent side effects?

- How can I manage the depression, grief, and anxiety that surround and infuse the cancer experience?

- What if there were simple techniques I could use to help release me from these negative emotions?

- Is there a way to hold onto who I was before embarking on this turbulent trip and emerge on the other side with my mind, body, and spirit intact?

So many patients survive cancer treatment but never recover from the process. Why is that? This book will help answer these questions and more.

Cancer and Energy Medicine: A Healing Journey details my journey with an extremely aggressive cancer and how I rode that tsunami with the help of energy medicine to not just survive, but thrive! Now, I want to share the tools, tips, and techniques I used to facilitate my journey. These exercises are intended to be used as a supplement to a traditional approach to cancer treatment, but they can also be used independently. They are simple and designed so that you or a loved one can do them at anytime, anywhere. The exercises delineated here are introductory, self-help techniques. Some of the names have been changed or the techniques have been adapted due to the limitations of this disease. If you are fortunate enough to have access to an Eden Energy Medicine (EEM) practitioner, you may find that they are trained in more advanced cancer energy medicine interventions, but those interventions are beyond the scope of this book.

What is Energy Medicine?

Energy medicine is an umbrella term that describes a wide range of modalities, including acupuncture, reiki, and yoga. As the name implies, it is based upon the understanding that energy predates form and accessing more subtle energy systems that exist in and around the body can positively impact one's health. All major cultural traditions and religions acknowledge, name, and work with these forces, but they might call it something different: chi, qi, prana, kundalini, the holy spirit, or life force. Science is beginning to measure some of these subtle frequencies, but most have yet to be assessed.[1]

The Eden Method is another modality that would be included under the energy medicine umbrella. What is the Eden Method and what makes it unique? Based upon the five element theory of Chinese medicine (TCM), the Eden Method is a system that puts the individual at the center of their own health. Traditional Western medicine views the patient as a passive bystander and it's the physician's job to "fix" the patient with drugs or surgery. The Eden Method turns this construct on its head and puts the individual at the center of their healing journey. It operates from the premise that the body is always seeking balance (homeostasis) and is designed to heal itself. Using simple holds or movement on or around the body, these subtle energy systems can begin to come back into balance. By partnering and communicating with our body's nine energy systems, we can take control of and responsibility for our health and help to heal ourselves. The Eden Method can be used as a support to traditional Western medical treatment or it can be a stand-alone healing method. In this book, the Eden Method is used as a means to support traditional Western medical care. (The terms Eden Method and EEM will be used interchangeably throughout this book.)

Just as the body's anatomy and physiology are complex and interdependent, so are its nine energy systems. Each plays a role independent of the other and yet, they are also connected and interdependent upon each other. These nine systems, in turn, interact with the body's physiological systems by means of the endocrine, circulatory, respiratory, immune, digestive, musculoskeletal, integumentary (skin, hair and nails), lymphatic, urinary, reproductive, and nervous systems. In *Cancer and Energy Medicine: A Healing Journey*, you will be working with most of the nine systems, but doing so does not require an in-depth understanding of what they are or how they operate.

These are the nine main energy systems:
- Meridians
- Aura or Biofield
- Chakras
- Electrics
- Celtic Weave

- Radiant Circuits
- Five Rhythms
- Triple Warmer
- Grid

For a more in-depth explanation of the nine energy systems, I recommend reading Donna Eden's book *Energy Medicine*: *Balance Your Body's Energies for Optimum Health, Joy, and Vitality*.[2]

Emotional Freedom Technique (EFT) is the other major energy medicine modality I used throughout my treatment. It is also based upon TCM and uses acupuncture points to help shift negative emotions or memories. We will explore EFT in this book, but there are also scores of EFT books and even more videos to be found on YouTube, so resources are plentiful.[3]

How to Use This Book

Cancer and Energy Medicine: A Healing Journey is divided into two parts. Part 1 details my cancer journey which included chemotherapy, surgery, and radiation. In Chapters 1 through 10, you will learn how I managed my trimodal cancer treatment, the obstacles I encountered, and how I overcame them. (Full disclosure: Part I is a no-holds-barred, brutally honest rendition that doesn't sugar-coat anything.) Although I used more than 30 alternative modalities during my ordeal[4], this book works with those in which I have an expertise: EEM and EFT. When referenced in Part I, energy medicine terms are bolded and cross-referenced to Part II where they are defined in greater depth.

Part ll brings hope and empowerment as you explore 40 exercises you can use to help navigate your journey. Chapter 11 explores energy medicine fundamentals that were critical to keep balanced throughout my treatment. Chapters 12–15 examine specific issues and side effects that arose during chemotherapy, surgery, radiation, and recovery. They detail the techniques and tools I used to manage each of them. Protocols that were lightly introduced in Part I are explained in greater detail in Part II. Energy medicine terms mentioned throughout the book are defined in the Glossary.

There is a fair amount of information in this book. If you are attempting to read it while undergoing cancer treatment, you may find it overwhelming at times. Rather than thinking you must do everything here, take it in bits and pieces. Reframe the process to be one of: I am beginning a relationship and communication with my body. Do what you can only when you feel up to it. Better yet, consider enlisting the help of a loved one. My cancer clients who had someone working on them did the best overall with their treatments. They love you and want to do something to help. Allowing them to do energy work on you empowers them and allows them to better support you through this process. They should do the exercises too; they'll need the benefits!

Part I

Dancing With Death

*In the Midst of Winter, I found there was inside me,
an Invincible Summer.*[5]

Albert Camus

Chapter 1

The Set Up

The spring of 2021 was an exciting time! The world was finally emerging from the COVID-19 lockdowns. My energy medicine practice was thriving, and I was teaching new practitioners the joys and rewards of this exciting healing modality. In addition, I was about to become a grandmother of two babies. Life was good and I was grateful. Yes, I had been working nonstop, six days a week for many years, but I was finally doing what I loved, so I didn't feel the need to rest. I hadn't been sick in more than a decade, and I felt invincible! When we weren't working, Jean-Pierre, my husband, and I flew to Massachusetts to spend time with our daughters, Kimberly and Nathalie, who were each due to give birth in May.

Remy and Wesley were born within a week of each other, May 6th and May 13th respectively, and I was on hand to help where I could. Both moms were breastfeeding, and both of them developed mastitis within a week of each other. As they dealt with the pain, I started to notice pain in my right breast. I laughed it off, telling myself that I was suffering from "sympathetic mastitis," but I scheduled a mammogram, nevertheless. I had to wait two weeks for the first available appointment, so I tried to ignore what I was feeling. This couldn't be breast cancer, I thought, because breast cancer doesn't develop overnight.

Over the next week, the breast started becoming redder, hotter, and more painful, so I decided to go to the local hospital emergency room. They diagnosed me with a breast infection, prescribed antibiotics, and referred me to a breast specialist at a Johns Hopkins affiliated hospital. I was relieved. The antibiotics seemed to help. The breast wasn't as painful, and it wasn't getting worse. Another week went by. I met with a breast specialist, who examined me and declared it was *granicular mastitis*—an extremely rare form of mastitis that can be painful and develop virtually overnight. She said to continue with the antibiotics for another week; if it hadn't cleared up by then, she would need to do surgery to clean it out.

Surgery? My mind started to race: "I can't have surgery! I'm an energy medicine practitioner. I hadn't taken a prescription drug in over a decade. Allergic reactions to medications are what landed me in the energy medicine world in the first place. I don't do traditional medicine!" Two weeks went by. My breast wasn't getting any better and I was developing an allergic reaction to the antibiotics. In fact, the breast was getting harder and more painful, and I was feeling pressure in my armpit. I was in enough pain that I started to become open to the possibility that surgery might be the best option because, whatever this was, I needed to get it out of my body—ASAP!

The surgeon scheduled surgery for the following Tuesday. Fortunately, one of the staff physicians intervened and insisted on a complete biopsy prior to surgery. We were in the full throes of the COVID-19 epidemic, so I had to go alone, but I figured I'd be done in an hour or two and bounce back to seeing clients the next day. Never having had a biopsy before, I had no idea what to expect, but what happened next was something I could never have imagined.

After they made the incision on my right breast, the pain was so excruciating, I couldn't move. I could only lay there and cry. The staff had never seen anything like this and didn't know what to make of it. When I asked for something to ease the pain, they said they couldn't give me anything because I wasn't an inpatient. (This would be the first of my many frustrations with the medical profession.) I was left alone in a cold, dark exam room. After several hours of lying on the table all alone in a heap of tears, I managed to scrape myself together and drive home.

On the Monday before Tuesday's surgery, the biopsy results came in: *invasive ductal carcinoma of the right breast and lymph nodes*. It was bad enough to hear that I had cancer, but it got worse: *inflammatory breast cancer* (IBC), *stage III*. What? Inflammatory breast cancer? I'd never even heard of it!

Acute inflammatory breast cancer, by definition, starts at stage III. Less than five percent of all breast cancers are this extremely rare type and are often misdiagnosed as breast mastitis. It is a complex cancer because it is actually a cancer of the lymphatic system and the skin that just happens to develop in the breast ducts. Since it develops via the lymph nodes, those must be removed in addition to the breast. Because it develops quickly (it can come on within a few weeks), it is already at stage III or IV when it's diagnosed. Until recently, five-year survival rates didn't go much past the 50th percentile. This is not a "wait and see" kind of tumor. People who forgo any of the trimodal treatments—chemotherapy, surgery, and radiation— can be dead within six months.

Treatment consists of six rounds of chemotherapy to try and shrink the tumor prior to surgery. Within three weeks of finishing chemo, a radical mastectomy is performed which includes removal of the entire breast and as much skin and adjacent lymph nodes as possible since IBC tends to return in the skin. Surgery is followed a few weeks later by 35 rounds of radiation to the entire torso, from the clavicle to the base of the rib cage. Radiation kills any microscopic cancer cells that might remain post-surgery. As a friend of mine who works as a nurse in breast oncology said, "IBC treatment is the most grueling of all breast cancer treatments."

But how did I get this? I spent the better part of two decades avoiding medical treatment of any kind. Moreover, I'd done time on "Hospital Row" and made it my life's mission to never go back there. Staring down this diagnosis, however, I was immediately transported back to Hospital Row.

To Hell and Back

It all began during the summer of 2002. Our son, Jonathan, was like any other eight-year-old boy: rambunctious, curious, and lots of fun. We noticed some bruising on his legs when he came back from swim practice one day, but assumed it was because he hit his leg while at the pool. When bruises started to show up on his torso a few days later, however, we became concerned. Jean-Pierre, a family physician, ordered blood tests. The results did not look good.

We scheduled an appointment with a pediatric oncologist, who looked at the results and referred us to Georgetown Hospital's Lombardi Cancer Center. Within 24 hours, we were given the diagnosis: *acute lymphatic leukemia*. Acute lymphatic leukemia is a blood cancer that starts in the bone marrow and affects the white blood cells. If not treated quickly, it will spread throughout the body.

Acute lymphatic leukemia? Our precious Jonathan? Our lives would never be the same again! After the initial shock wore off, we learned that Jon's treatment would consist of three and a half years of chemotherapy along with many hospitalizations and multiple spinal taps. We adjusted our schedules so I would stay with Jonathan whenever he had inpatient treatments. Fortunately, we caught the cancer early, so he wasn't considered high risk, and he went into remission within a couple of months. Survival rates for childhood leukemia at that time were at about 75%, so we had hope. Despite those encouraging numbers, the next several years would be arduous. Jonathan would not be able to go to school, participate in sports, or do other activities a child his age would enjoy. Nearly every time we went to the hospital, he would receive a spinal tap, a procedure that involved removing a cerebral fluid sample from the spine.

Watching my child undergo this procedure on a regular basis was painful, but witnessing the side effects from the chemotherapy was much worse. After a few months of receiving a drug called vincristine, Jon developed such bad foot drop, he couldn't walk. He would cry out in pain at night because the drug was causing leg cramps. There is nothing worse as a parent than watching your child suffer and being powerless to do anything to stop it. Out of desperation to help ease his pain, I studied foot reflexology. Every night, I would massage Jon's feet so he could sleep. Once, when we were watching *The Wizard of Oz* while he was getting an infusion, Jonathan had a heart attack. Another drug made him temporarily blind. His reactions were so rare, the doctors had to go to the medical books to confirm that they were drug-related side effects.

Despite those rare side effects, nothing compares to what happened on January 21, 2003, when Jon's oncologist informed us that after 18 months of treatment, Jon's cancer had returned—this time in his cerebral spinal fluid. This was highly unusual and meant he would not survive without a transplant of some kind. A transplant would require a bone marrow or stem cell donor. It would also require radiation of Jon's entire body. Total body radiation can cause brain damage. In addition to digesting this shocking news, we were now facing two new obstacles: finding a donor who was a match for Jon and keeping him in remission until he could undergo a transplant. Without a good match, his chances of long-term survival were nil.

The nights I spent at the hospital trying to stay positive and watching happy movies took an abrupt 180-degree turn. I spent countless hours on the internet, which was still in its infancy at the time, searching for which hospitals had the best transplant survival rates and whether a stem cell or a bone marrow transplant might be a better choice.

I scoured medical journals until the wee hours of the morning, trying to make sense of what I could in between medical terms I did not understand. I contacted the best pediatric oncology departments in the country to find out what drugs and radiation dosages they used for transplants. I was surprised to learn that not every hospital was using the same drugs and, more importantly, the same dosage of radiation.

I concluded that I needed to become my son's best advocate and question everything I heard. As I toured pediatric oncology departments, I witnessed transplant survivors who appeared to suffer brain damage due to the amount of radiation they had received. I began to realize that survival was not the only critical issue we faced; long-term quality of life became as important as survivorship.

Expect a Miracle

With this huge setback, I knew we couldn't rely solely on ourselves to fight this battle. Yes, Jean-Pierre was a physician and I was a lawyer, so we had skills that served us well in trying to negotiate the process, but we needed to rely on a "Higher Power" to help us make the right decisions, as these were now life-and-death matters. I created a huge sign and hung it on the wall opposite Jon's hospital bed so we would see it first thing in the morning. It read: *Expect a Miracle* in big, bold colors. The "miracle" I was seeking wasn't that the cancer would disappear; the miracle would be that we could successfully navigate the landmine–filled road of potential complications, errors, or setbacks to achieve long-term survival.

The first order of business was to keep Jon in remission and find a donor. Sadly, many people wait years and never find a donor. Next, we had to find the best place for Jon's transplant. Between January 21st and March 15th, we managed to keep Jon in remission: *Miracle #1*. Then we tested our two daughters, Kim who was 16 years old at the time and Nathalie, who was 14. Kim turned out to be a perfect match for Jon. It was as if they were cut from the same cloth - a true rarity as only 25% of transplant patients have a sibling match. *Miracle #2.*

Then, at the end of March, our oncologists told us Jon's cancer had returned. My husband and I prayed a prayer of resignation that we had done all that we could to keep our precious boy alive, but it was not part of the plan for him to survive. Two days later, the doctors said the test was a false positive; in fact, Jon was still in remission. *Miracle #3.*

The post-relapse treatment was brutal. They kept Jon in remission by doubling his chemotherapy. He was in a wheelchair. Due to his low blood counts, he contracted every op-portunistic disease in the hospital, from *C difficile* to *staph aureus*. There were times he was so sick that we didn't think he would survive whatever infection it was he was fighting. But he did: *Miracle #4.*

We had one last obstacle to overcome: finding the best place for Jon's transplant. This proved more challenging than I could ever have imagined. First came the decision as to which was better: a stem cell or a bone marrow transplant? Kim, the donor, was an aspiring professional dancer, and taking bone marrow from her hip could jeopardize her future career. This tipped the scales in favor of a stem cell transplant, but stem cell transplants were new at the time, and very few hospitals were doing them. In fact, the five-year, long-term survival rates at some of the institutions doing stem cell transplants were less than 17%. Despite those statistics, hospitals could earn up to a $1 million per stem cell transplant, so we needed to carefully weigh the institutions' financial interest with what was in our son's best interest.

A friend suggested I investigate the National Institutes of Health (NIH) to see if they had any studies for relapsed leukemia patients. Many people think of the NIH as a place of last resort, particularly in the case of cancer, but I knew it was also a place of innovative research that would one day trickle down to become what is known as the "standard of care" in medical institutions throughout the world. Combing through the NIH website late one night, I found a stem cell transplant study at the National Heart, Lung and Blood Institute (NHLBI) that seemed to match Jon's diagnosis.

This study was unique for several reasons. In a standard stem cell or bone marrow transplant, the donor's blood is extracted through the hip bone, the red cells are discarded and the stem cells are retained for the recipient. This approach can create problems for the donor such as anemia or pain at the site of extraction, but there is also some risk to the recipient if a virus or other bacteria is present. Moreover, in a traditional transplant, no white cells are extracted from the donor and up to 2400 rads of total body radiation is considered to be normal. In this study, the donor's blood was extracted through a catheter on the inner thigh, every cell was counted, any viruses or bacteria were removed, both the donor's stem cells and white cells were retained and the red blood cells were returned to the donor. They then transplanted a combination of the stem cells and white cells to the patient. Transplanting both the red and white stem cells gave the recipient a better chance of adapting to the transplant without triggering too much graft versus host disease, a reaction patients can have when their body rejects the new stem cells. Even better, this study used half as much radiation as what was considered the standard of care in hospital treatments. It was state-of-the-art medical care, and its survival rate was 87%! *Miracle # 5.* There was just one caveat: Patients had to be a minimum of ten years old to participate in the study. It was April and Jon would not turn ten until June 21st.

For the first time, I felt hope that I had found the absolute best place for Jon's treatment. I had to go against doctors' advice and even had to fight to get an appointment at the NHLBI, but when I did, the doctor heading up the study agreed that Jon met all the criteria. Now, it was a matter of keeping him in remission for another two months. On June 21st, Jon was accepted into the study and on July 13th, he received his sister's stem cells. *Miracle #6.*

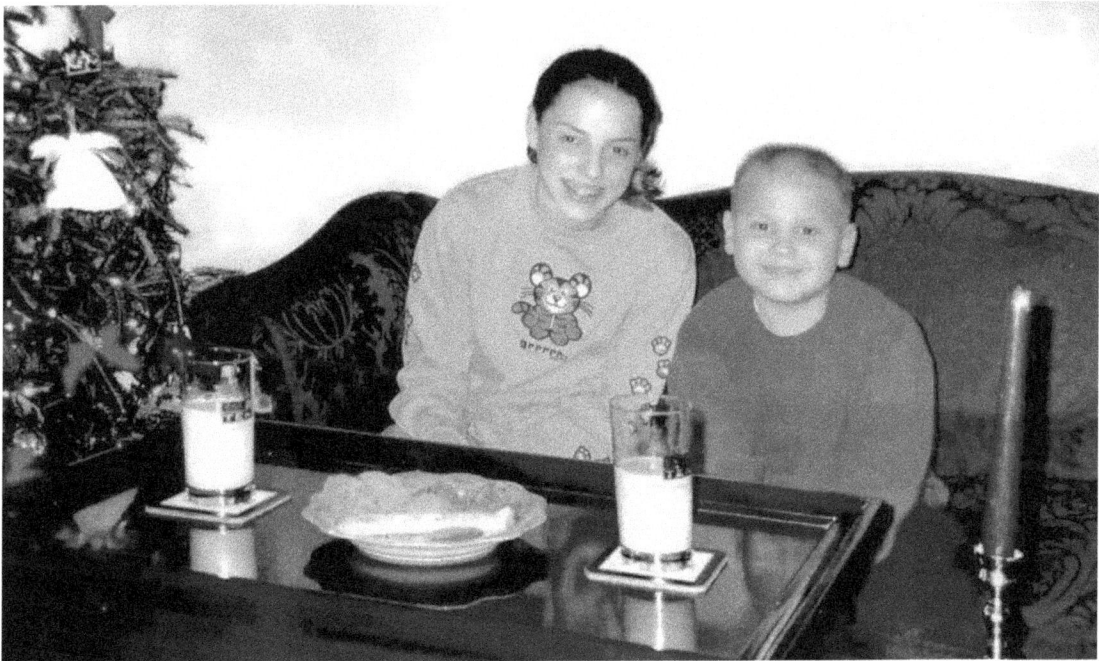

Kimberly and Jonathan

The miracles I wished for on that March day didn't end there. We witnessed many other miracles over the course of Jon's treatment. The love and support of neighbors who organized dinners for us month after month. Prayer circles organized by friends and families from a host of different religious and cultural backgrounds. Each played a role; each had an impact in saving Jon's life. That was 20 years ago. The boy who couldn't walk or run like other children is now a professional writer, dance teacher, and coach. Getting a lower dose of radiation allowed Jon to graduate from college at 20 years old and go on to have a successful career. Long-term, late effects from chemo or issues like graft-versus-host disease never materialized. As we walked the arduous path together during those three years, I would continually hear these words: "Yea, though I walk through the valley of the shadow of death, I will fear no evil; For you are with me; your rod and your staff, they comfort me."

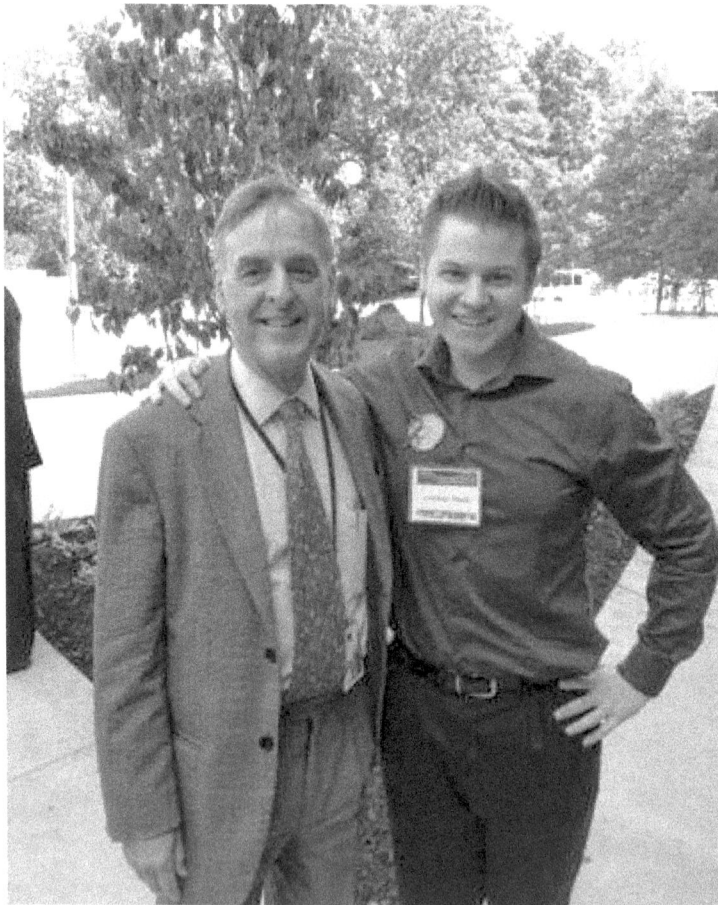

Dr. Barrett and Jonathan

Picking Up the Pieces

Fighting the battle to keep Jon alive came with a price: my own health. I had suffered from chronic health issues most of my adult life: lower back pain, irritable bowel syndrome, headaches, sinusitis, and allergies. As I entered menopause, however, everything accelerated. As soon as I stepped out of bed in the morning, I would have shooting pains throughout my joints. I had severe insomnia and my hair was falling out in hunks. I was allergic to nearly all medications, including allergy medications. I couldn't walk upstairs because every joint in my body hurt. As much as I wanted to, I couldn't work because I was in so much pain.

I was first diagnosed with hypothyroidism and then a combination of rheumatoid arthritis, skin lupus, and connective tissue disease. I called it "Autoimmune Disease of the Month" because I never knew how or when it would manifest. It would morph from my skin to my joints to my back. Coincidentally, I was the same age my father was when he was diagnosed with Parkinson's disease. I vividly recall watching him deteriorate over the next 20 years, spending his last five years in a wheelchair, unable to speak. I didn't want that to be my future.

Although this was a wake-up call for me, I was between a rock and a hard place. If I went the traditional medicine route, I would be on medication for the rest of my life, but my body was allergic to most medications. I needed to find something else—something I could do that didn't involve drugs and didn't require me to constantly get "fixed" by someone else every few weeks.

The answer to my prayer was stumbling upon a YouTube video of Donna Eden. "Who was this woman?" I wondered. She was older than me, but she had the kind of energy of which I could only dream. What was she talking about? Nothing she said made any sense, but whatever it was she had, I wanted some!

That evening, I went to a friend's house, and there on the coffee table was the book *Energy Medicine: Balance Your Body's Energies for Optimum Health, Joy, and Vitality*, by Donna Eden. Believing there are no such things as coincidences in life, I took this as a sign; I needed to explore EEM further. I discovered she was teaching at a conference the following weekend in New Jersey, so without a second thought, I drove to New Jersey. By the end of the weekend, I discovered how to heal my lower back pain which had plagued me for decades—even surgery hadn't helped. I was hooked. I needed to study with Donna Eden!

Over the course of the next several years, Jean-Pierre and I traveled to Arizona to learn all we could about the Eden Method. Initially less enthusiastic than I, Jean-Pierre eventually had his own up close and personal experience with energy medicine and became a believer too. Within several months, my joint pain disappeared, my hair was growing back, and I was sleeping better. By the end of the first year, I had more energy and less pain than I could ever have imagined. For the first time in my life, I wasn't afraid to grow old.

Shifting Gears

It had been years since I had practiced law full-time. I sat on a couple of boards, but I was too sick to work. With these new developments, however, I was able to move forward with a career I had to previously forego. I had no intention of having an energy medicine practice for several reasons. My own health was too vulnerable and I had no medical education or training. I had spent the last two decades wanting to practice law again, and I was not at an age when one could easily switch careers. Besides, why did I spend all that time, effort, and money on law school if I didn't practice? While it was true that I had a passion for EEM—it was fun and truly made a difference in people's lives—how could I make a career change at my age? Not to mention the huge ego-stroking benefit of introducing myself as an attorney instead of a "witch doctor." So, armed with my newfound health, I started working at a local law firm practicing real estate law.

Knowing the benefits of energy medicine, Jean-Pierre would periodically ask me to see one of his patients who had not been helped with traditional medicine. Typically, all the requisite tests had been done without revealing the cause of the illness, or the medications weren't working. Nevertheless, I resisted. There was a reason I used to call my husband "The Carrier"; I was always battling whatever cold or virus he had seen in his office that day. The last thing I needed was to see his patients at his office!

Months passed. As my energies continued to get stronger, the glittering, shiny seduction of the legal profession began to fade. The work was stressful and tedious, but I pushed through, thinking: "This is what I'm trained to do." My enthusiasm for EEM didn't fade, however, so I found myself helping my boss and staff members with whatever health issues they were encountering. I started to realize that I genuinely loved doing the energy work and the legal work was just a paycheck.

The tipping point came when a staff member, "Julie," injured her back while walking down some steps. Her back was in severe spasm and she couldn't move. Someone called 911. Our staff gingerly placed her onto a table to wait for an ambulance. Julie, however, was adamant that she didn't want to go to the hospital. One minute she was screaming from the pain, the next minute, she was crying because she didn't want to go to the hospital.

Out of desperation, my boss called me down from my office to see if I could do anything to help ease Julie's pain and anxiety until the medics arrived. Using energy medicine, I immediately sedated the meridian which governs stress response and the one related to her lower back pain. Over the course of the next several minutes, Julie's anxiety abated and she was able to move a little. I continued doing this for about the next 15 minutes. By the time the ambulance arrived, Julie was standing up and smiling. The medics checked her out and said she didn't need to go to the hospital after all.

That was a pivotal moment for me to consider that, yes, perhaps I could do this work full-time. First, though, I would need some kind of healthcare license because I had no formal medical training and without a license, my right to practice could be revoked at any time. Since time wasn't on my side, I needed to do something fast, and with Jon in his sophomore year at Georgetown University, I needed to do something that wouldn't break the bank either. I decided to enroll in massage therapy school.

For the next year, I went to school in the morning, worked at my law firm in the afternoon, and saw clients at night. It didn't bother me that I was working long hours—I was happy to be working again, but this time with something I loved. When I made the final jump into full-time energy work, I was working seven days a week and loving every minute. I was never sick, and all my previous illnesses and symptoms were gone. I had reversed my hypothyroidism. My back pain was nonexistent. My autoimmune issues resolved. I had the best head of hair I had ever had in my life. I leapt out of bed every morning ready to seize the day!

Back to Square One

When COVID-19 hit, life slowed down for several months, but then the pace picked up a bit. By the end of October 2020, I was back to seeing clients. By this time, I had taken additional training and was teaching future EEM practitioners, many of whom were also my clients. Unfortunately, my self-care slowed significantly due to COVID-19. I wasn't getting energy work or massage. I was teaching four-day, ten-hour classes and not taking a break before seeing clients. I was working six days a week. When I wasn't working, I was traveling to Massachusetts to spend time with my children and grandchildren. Although I felt fine, I noticed after I had the COVID-19 vaccine, I started to develop odd viral infections, including shingles and strange sores in my mouth that wouldn't go away. A month later, my breast blew up.

Dark Night of the Soul

Cancer? I had cancer? Day by day, it started to sink in. I had to close my practice immediately and say good-bye to my clients, whom I genuinely loved. It was as if a bomb had dropped, and, just as with Jonathan, my life would never be the same. The official diagnosis was on July 17th, but my first round of chemo wasn't scheduled until August 1st. I read up on the aggressive nature of this cancer and was terrified that, over the course of the next three weeks, it would morph from stage III and stage IV because so much time was passing. I could feel my lymph nodes swelling. I spent my days and nights doing EEM on myself to try and hold off that possibility.

Even though I had been down this path with Jonathan, it was different this time. I was a caregiver and bystander then; it was not my body that was undergoing the treatment. This time, I was concerned about how my body would handle the chemo because I couldn't even take over-the-counter medications:

How would I manage multiple rounds of infusions and blood tests when I'm triggered at the sight of a needle?

How would my age impact my ability to manage what was coming my way?

Even if I survived the chemo, surgery, and radiation, what would my long-term quality of life look like?

On the other hand, I had some amazing tools in my arsenal I didn't have when Jonathan was sick. My background in energy medicine put me light-years ahead of where I was when all I could do was foot reflexology. The question was: How could I use my energy medicine tools to help me get through what would be a harrowing journey? EEM saved my health once: was it enough to get me through this ordeal?

I knew that just because I was an EEM practitioner, it didn't mean that I would have an easier time than other patients. In fact, due to my autoimmune history, I knew that I would be the patient who would have the odd side effects others didn't. There was no way I could continue to work and I wasn't the type to put on a happy face and pretend all was well.

Although I tried to find ways to rationalize why I didn't need the poison/slash/burn approach to my tumor, I knew that forgoing any of those options with an IBC diagnosis was a death sentence. I was being forced to face all three treatments head-on with the hope that EEM could help me navigate this razor-sharp tightrope without falling off or fatally cutting myself.

Chapter 2

The Poisoning

Round One: July 31, 2021

The Battles Begin

With my medical history in mind, I met with the oncologist to review my biopsy results. I was so overwhelmed; I broke down in tears. I sobbed as I told him my medical history and how I couldn't take medications like other people. I shared my story of how I discovered EEM and healed my autoimmune issues. I went on to explain that I specialized in helping cancer clients and their caregivers get through chemo, surgery, and radiation with the help of energy medicine. (How ironic: Just a couple of years before, I was teaching breast cancer patients and their families the benefits of energy medicine at Johns Hopkins Hospital in Baltimore, MD, and here I was at one of their satellite offices with breast cancer.) I told him I needed to *energy test* the medication that was going to be used so I could know which energy systems it affected.

He must have taken pity on me because he gave me permission to energy test the medication before receiving the infusions. This was no easy task. These medications are so toxic that anyone administering them has to be gowned up. Even though I was given permission to energy test the substance, I knew it would test toxic, so I decided to see what I could do to counteract the side effects.

How to Energy Self-Test

Energy testing is a biofeedback mechanism that conveys information about the body. There are many ways to energy test, but the simplest way is to self-test. The body will reveal the truth if you ask it in the proper way. Using the body as a pendulum, you can discover the truth by understanding whether your body is attracted to or repelled by something.

You will need to be standing for this exercise. It's easy for your mind to interfere with your testing, so you will need to start with a 'baseline' test to make sure your answers are accurate.

1. While standing, take an inhale through your nose and an exhale through your mouth.

2. At the bottom of your exhale, state your name out loud: "My name is _____."

3. Notice if your body moves forwards or backwards after you make the statement. It should move forward if it is a true statement.

4. Now take an inhale through your nose and an exhale through your mouth and state a name that is clearly not your name, like: "My name is Sponge Bob."

5. Your body should move backwards since this is a false statement.

6. You are now ready to ask your body a question.

7. You want to ask a question that has to do with your physical health, for example, whether a food or supplement is beneficial for you or whether an organ needs help. (Only licensed healthcare providers can energy test a medication dosage.)

8. Place the food or substance you wish to test at your solar plexus, just above your navel.

9. Now using your body as a pendulum, ask your body a specific question and see whether your body moves forwards or backwards.

NOTE: This technique is taught in greater detail on Page 121.

Drip, Drip, Drip

My chemotherapy infusion was administered outpatient over the course of about five hours. Once I had the TCHP cocktail (Taxotere, Carboplatin, Herceptin, and Perjeta), I taught my nurse how to energy test. (She was a holistic nurse and knew a bit about energy medicine, so she was thrilled to learn more about it.) I balanced the meridians that were reacting to the chemotherapy so my body would not react with shock or weakness in the face of the medications. Just doing these simple things allowed me to have some sense of power over the process and calmed my body's stress response.

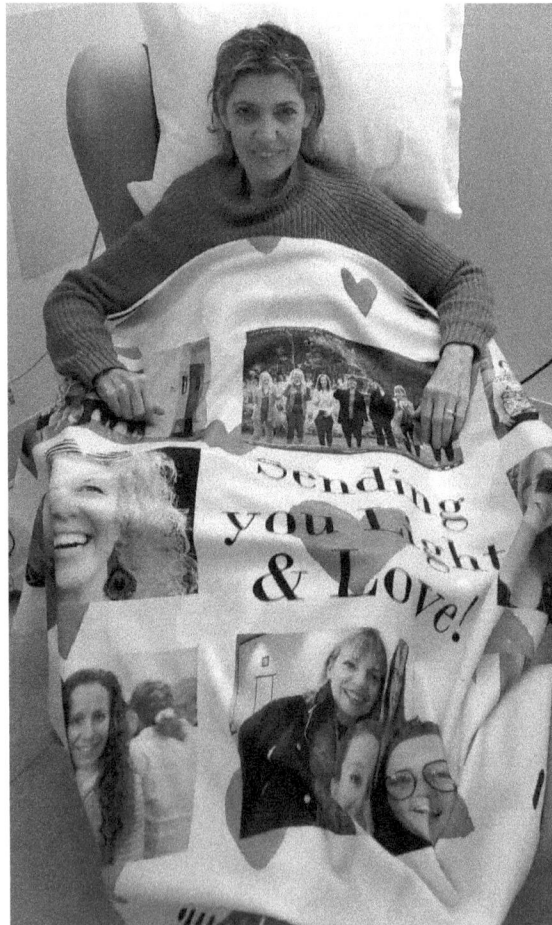

Wrapping myself in a blanket my students created helped me feel better.

Even though COVID-19 was everywhere, I was allowed to have one person with me at all times. One of my students, Heather, was kind enough to come to the hospital and performed an acupressure protocol on me while I was getting my infusions. She also *cleared my chakras* to help move toxins out of my field.

How to Clear Chakras

1. Imagine there is a clock superimposed on the recipient's body. The twelve is at the head and the six is at the feet.
2. Starting at the root chakra, make counterclockwise circles very slowly for several minutes about four inches off the body in line with each of the seven chakras. (See photo on Page 133).
3. Do this for several minutes.
4. End with making clockwise circles for about thirty seconds.
5. Move up the body to each chakra and do the same thing, making counterclockwise circles for several minutes and then clockwise circles for about one minute.
6. Do not make clockwise circles over the part of the body that has the tumor.

NOTE: This technique is taught in greater detail on Page 132.

I was doing pretty well until the nurse administering the Taxotere missed my vein and the medication leaked into my arm. It was an extremely toxic drug so when this happened, it was as if my arm had been set on fire. It was the first of my many battle scars to come.

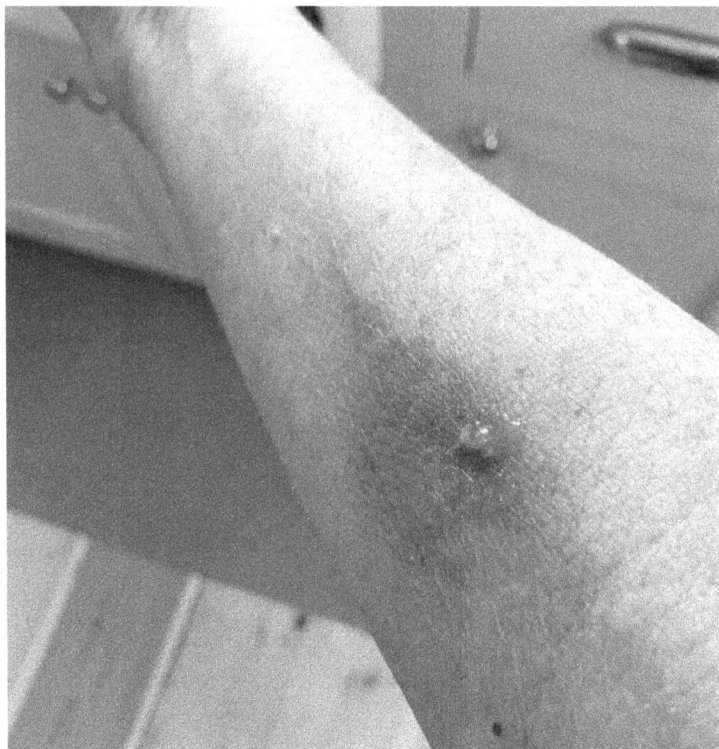

A Crash Landing

I didn't know what to expect from the chemo's side effects, even though my son had endured it for more than a year. This was a different diagnosis with different drugs and a different body. The doctors at Johns Hopkins warned me I had a 48-hour window to do what I needed to do before the side effects would set in. On the one hand, I was relieved that the ticking time bomb in my chest had been stopped and I managed to remain at stage III, but I decided it would be better for me to be treated nearer to where my daughters lived. So on the day after receiving my first round of chemo and hopped up on steroids, I boarded a plane and flew to Massachusetts.

I knew it would be tough, but no one could have prepared me for what happened next. The plane didn't crash, but I did. I woke up the next day and couldn't move my head off the pillow. It was as if I was glued to the mattress. I'd never experienced anything like this before. I had no appetite, and the only time I could move was to go to the bathroom because diarrhea had already set in. Despite my best intentions, I certainly couldn't do any energy medicine to help myself.

I was nauseous and there were sores developing in my mouth that were extremely painful. I had been taking Imodium to stave off the diarrhea, but I seemed to have developed an allergic reaction to it because I had a rash on my neck and torso. I couldn't talk or eat. My friends who came to help made me rice and soup, but I couldn't eat because of the mouth sores. Nothing tasted good. I couldn't even drink water. Seeing the shape I was in, Jean-Pierre went to the drugstore and brought back a dizzying array of over-the-counter medications for diarrhea, gas, indigestion, heartburn, and pain to try and help alleviate my side effects.

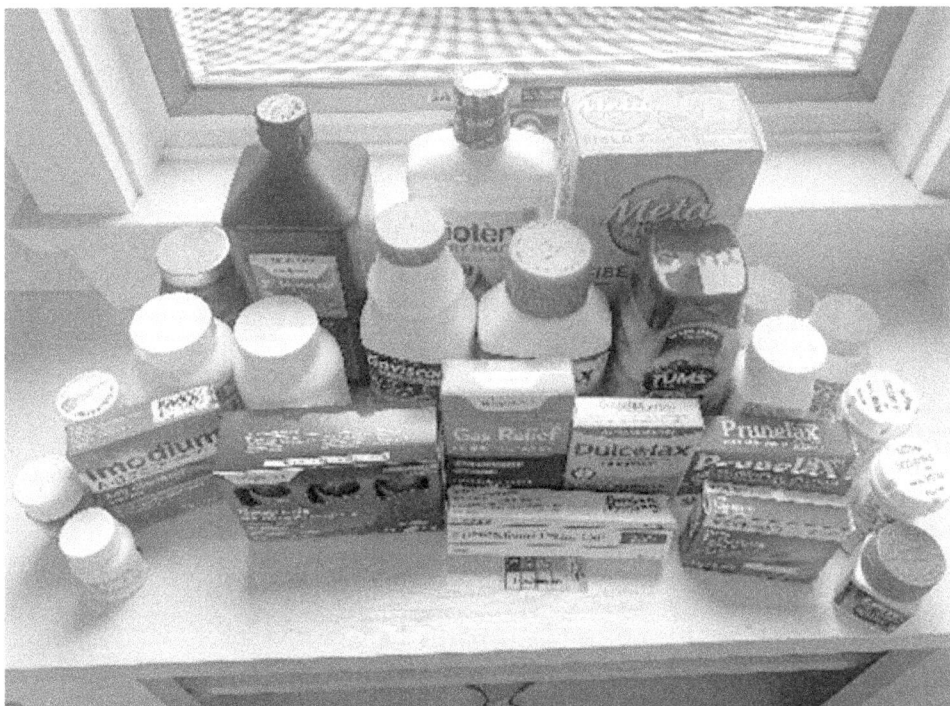

As someone who prided herself on never needing prescription or over-the-counter medications, I would be making up for all the lost time and was about to enter a world I knew nothing about. I could see it was going to be a roller-coaster ride.

By the next day, my mouth sores were in full bloom, and it felt like I was getting cut with a knife every time I swallowed. The sores took up residence on the sides of the throat, underneath my tongue, and along the edges of my lower lip. I did my online research and discovered that the ones on the edge of the mouth were called *cheilitis* and were secondary to chemo and a weakened immune system.

Oil pulling, an Ayurvedic technique that involves swishing, but not swallowing, oil in your mouth to kill harmful bacteria seemed to help, so there was some relief from the constant stabbing pain, but it only got worse if I tried to eat or drink. I forced myself to eat tiny amounts of rice, soup, or applesauce, but between the sores and nausea, I couldn't even keep water down.

As the days passed, my strength returned a bit, so I was able to walk around with the help of walking sticks. The rash from my allergic reaction to Imodium had been slowly creeping up my neck, down my arms, and along my torso. It was hot, burning, and itchy. I stopped taking the Imodium, so it didn't get worse, but then I risked having my diarrhea return. Sure enough, within a few hours, it made its reappearance.

By Day Five, I was so miserable, I was operating at the pace of a four-month-old. I knew this because I had two four-month-olds to compare myself to: Wesley and Remy. I slept, woke up, ate insignificant amounts of food, got indigestion, went potty, rested from having gone potty, ate, got stomach pain from the digestive process, went potty again, rested, ate—and the same vicious cycle started all over again. At least no one had to change my diaper - yet!

By the end of the week, I was doing much better. I was no longer nauseous, and my bowels seemed to have settled down. My rash, cuts, and sores appeared to be slowly healing, and my energy level was coming back. I still hadn't moved out of the bed or my pajamas much, though. It felt good to feel more like myself rather than being locked in a zombie's body. I kept trying to find a way to describe how chemo felt. The best analogy I could think of was: Close your eyes and imagine you're a zombie. Now imagine you're a sick zombie. That's what having chemo felt like.

On August 12th, I met my Boston oncologist for the first time. I was so weak, my husband had to push me in a wheelchair—after just one round of chemo! The oncologist looked at me and asked me why I was so weak. She asked if I was taking Imodium and I told her I was allergic to it. I filled her in on my autoimmune history, sharing that I was allergic to many medications and didn't require full dosages for my body to feel the effects of a medication. She said she would not adjust the dosage of any chemo because IBC is so aggressive. If I couldn't take the standard chemotherapy, she said, I would have to go on a drug called the "Red Devil" (doxorubicin).

Defrosting the Past

Like many cancer patients, I purchased every cancer book I could find. Some were focused on diet and metabolism, others on emotions. I read as many as possible because I knew they all contained a kernel of truth I could use to heal myself. I noticed that ever since I was diagnosed, my dreams had been stressful and I would wake up exhausted. As an EEM practitioner, I knew imbalanced emotions often underlie physical or mental issues. I was willing to examine every aspect of my mind or body's underlying terrain to see if I could begin to piece together what caused this phenomena.

I enlisted the help of one of my colleagues, Heather (a different Heather), to see if we could get to the root of some of these underlying emotional blockages. A psychotherapist, Heather was also trained in EEM. Her background allowed her to weave together energy medicine, imagery and something called *parts work*[6]. Even though we were working remotely, I was able to enter a deeply relaxed state so I could communicate with my meridians, organs, and other energy systems. This produced a profound level of awareness of what underlying issues might have been the soil through which my cancer could have grown. As we dialogued with these parts, I was transported to a time and place when I felt hopeless and helpless.

It was at Georgetown Hospital and I was walking in the hallway between my son's hospital room and the Lombardi Cancer Center. I had just learned that Jonathan, who had been diagnosed with acute lymphatic leukemia six months earlier, relapsed while on chemotherapy. The shock of that news was so overwhelming that some part of me could not process it. I was traumatized to my core. Using parts work, Heather helped me to dialogue with this frozen aspect of myself and let her know that my son fully recovered and went on to live a happy life. We were able to transport that frozen aspect of my personality out of the hospital hallway and allow her to integrate with my current "Self". We also helped her to release herself of guilt, self-blame, and shame around her responsibility as a mother to save her son's life.

While processing this memory, an image of my current grandsons came into view. The near-simultaneous births of my two male grandchildren somehow triggered that earlier traumatic memory in my subconscious. The awesome responsibility of bringing a new life into the world and wanting to protect and provide for them is a natural part of a parent's heart, but that part of my heart had been stuck and frozen in the traumatic memory and couldn't move forward. Heather's gentle coaching technique helped me to heal that aspect of myself and integrate the frozen memory.

Coming Down the Back Stretch

By the time I was two weeks out from Round One, my intestines had finally settled down. Whoever said the gut biome is the key to good health wasn't kidding. Without a smooth flow of nutrients through the alimentary canal, it's difficult to feel healthy or happy. My other nagging issues of mouth sores and the skin rash were also slowly resolving. I felt like I should have more energy, but I didn't really. I still felt sluggish and tired. I noticed there was only one problem when I started to feel better - I could feel the cancer coming back!

My next chemo round was in a few days. Although I was finally feeling better, my sense of normalcy also brought with it a sense of urgency:

- What did I need to do to prepare myself for this next round?
- What had I forgotten to anticipate so I could mount a response to what would happen on Friday?
- What did I need to accomplish before I wouldn't be able to function?

To complicate matters, I was scheduled to have port placement surgery the following day. Just the thought of it sent chills down my spine. For me, a port somehow represented the worst aspects of cancer: my powerlessness over my own body and becoming dependent on a manufactured device. On the one hand, it was a badge of shame that my body had failed me and I had to resort to outside forces to keep me alive. On the other hand, it would keep me from getting burned, preserve my veins, and cause me less pain in the long run. Those were comforting thoughts, and I held onto them, but adding a port also triggered my memory of Jonathan's Hickman line—his central venous catheter—which I had to flush every day. Whenever I see the scar on his chest, it's a vivid reminder of our ordeal.

Fortunately, I had tools to help me reframe the issue. To counteract my fears, I did *temporal tapping* to help prepare my body for what was to come. Even though I was starting the process a little late, I tapped in the following statements:

My body will have no problem integrating this port.
This port will be a welcome addition to my body.

Temporal Tapping

1. Start by making a goal: What is it that you want to achieve? For example, if you have a fear of needles, your goal might be that you can have a blood draw without feeling nauseous or faint.

2. Choose two statements that reflect your goal. Both should be positive, but one must have a negative word in it. Using our example of a fear of needles, one statement could be:
   I am not afraid of needles.
   The other statement might be:
   It's easy for me to have a blood draw.

3. By tapping these statements along the meridian line that governs the emotional brain, you can begin to shift entrenched habits.

4. Starting at your temple, tap the 'negative' statement on the **left** side of your head from your temple to behind your ear and down towards your neck while saying the statement out loud.

5. Say the statement five times out loud while tapping from your temple to your neck.

6. Do the same thing on your right side tapping in the 'positive' statement from your **right** temple to behind your ear five times.

7. Tap on both sides of your head while making these statements out loud at least five times a day so your body can begin to incorporate the new thought pattern.

NOTE: This technique is taught in greater detail on Page 125.

Accessing My Equity Account

Someone in an IBC support group said that having port placement surgery was the least difficult thing about their entire breast cancer journey, but I beg to differ. I hadn't had a surgical procedure in 20 years, so the thought of having my body cut open was an adjustment. The only available appointment was at 6 AM so as I sat waiting for the surgery center to open, I remembered my years on hospital duty, reliving all the procedures that Jonathan went through and knowing that complications could and did occur. Many people had been praying for us at that time, and I knew from my experience with Jonathan that this energy was a kind of energetic equity I could draw upon in times of need—a spiritual bank account, if you will. Knowing all the possible complications that might ensue, I decided to draw on that equity account and ask for things to go smoothly and without incident.

On my trip to the operating room, I was placed in an elevator with a young man on my left and a middle-aged man on my right. The three of us were taken downstairs to a floor that housed the surgical center. We were placed in stations next to each other, separated by a curtain on either side. I couldn't see them, but I could hear them. I learned quickly that they both were being treated for cancer. One had a blood infusion earlier in the week, and the other was off to get more chemo after this port placement. I was grateful that I could just go home and rest. Although I had been preparing my body with energy work, as I sat there waiting to meet my nurse, every cell in my body wanted to run. Rather than resist, however, I knew I had to stop and go with the flow; fighting would be futile. I could only move forward having faith that everything would work out as it should.

As I lay there, I listened as the man across from me had to deal with a doctor who somehow never took the course "Bedside Manners" in medical school. I listened while the nurse on the other side of me had to poke the sweet young man numerous times, but still couldn't find a vein. Accessing my equity account, I asked whomever I got would be wise and competent. Both of my wishes were granted. Mary, my nurse, was so adept at placing the IV that I didn't feel it go in at all and the physician assistant who would be doing the procedure was at least as old as I was, with deep wisdom and compassionate eyes.

Even with their combined experience and competence, the nurse and physician's assistant were both surprised at my early battle scars. Neither had ever seen a burn like the one on my arm, or my neck rash. The good news is they decided to place the port in my arm instead of my chest, so I considered that a win. Once they put the mask on my face to sedate me, I was out like a light and felt nothing after that. Why can't they do that when they give you chemo?

Calling on My Angels

The day after my surgery, I felt hung over from the sedative I had been given the day before. I was in pain from the incision and the skin rash. I was feeling overwhelmed and sad. I didn't usually feel this way, so I knew my energies had to be off. Sure enough, they were *homolateral*. I found the strength to make the correction. After about five minutes, I felt more hopeful, less pain, and had a greater degree of energy.

Correcting a Homolateral Pattern

1. Start by tapping your right hand to your right knee and your left hand to your left knee as if you were marching in place. Do this ten times.
2. Tap your right hand to your left knee and your left hand to your right knee. Do this ten times.
3. Repeat Steps 1 and 2 two more times: ten parallel and ten crossovers. Be sure to cross the midline of your body when you do the crossover tapping so your body gets the clear message that its energies need to start crossing over.
4. End with ten more crossover taps on each side of the body. This final set of crossover taps is what reinforces the message you want to give the body to stay crossed over.
5. Do these exercises several times a day if possible until your body can hold the pattern.

NOTE: This technique is taught in greater detail on Page 105.

I had completed only one round of chemo and I was in full Sick Zombie mode. There was a burn mark on my arm, a nasty-looking rash on my upper chest and neck, a huge hematoma on my upper arm from the port surgery, and I looked like I had aged ten years in five weeks. I thought about the breast cancer patients I saw when I taught at Johns Hopkin's Breast Cancer Center in Baltimore, MD. They were frail, worn down, and exhausted. And they were young! I was almost 65 years old and I didn't know if my body had the resiliency to bounce back from this. It was dawning on me that it was not just about whether I would survive, but how resilient would I be? Could my body withstand the relentless attacks it would be encountering? How could I keep my body in balance despite the onslaught coming its way? Maintaining healthy energetic patterns takes an effort even in the best of circumstances. Fortunately, I had two aces in my back pocket: my daughters. Nathalie was a nurse and Kimberly was an EEM practitioner. With them by my side, I was in good hands, and their help would prove to be invaluable throughout this trial.

Chapter 3

The Poisoning

Chemo Round 2: August 20, 2021

A Watershed Moment

I was in good shape going into this round because Kim insisted I have a massage beforehand and I had another remarkable energy medicine session with Heather. That was fortunate because I wasn't prepared for what happened when I arrived at the hospital. My hospital's infusion center consisted of large rooms containing six chairs separated by curtains. Despite Boston being in the throes of COVID-19, my neighbors were just a few feet away from me. The woman across the room had started her infusion about a half-hour before me. It sounded as though she and I were on the same regime, getting Taxotere for the same length of time. She was significantly younger than I and appeared to be doing well, laughing and talking with her companion who settled her in and then left to go back to work. Suddenly, I heard loud noises and saw nurses running into her room. She had gone into anaphylactic shock! At one point, there had to be close to fifteen medical staff in her small space. Fortunately, she was revived and wheeled out of the room.

A few minutes later, the woman next to me started vomiting violently. I listened in disbelief as the nurse told her there was nothing more they could do for her. She was miserable as she continued to vomit for what felt like an eternity. From witnessing this, I realized how lucky I was to have so many energy tools at my disposal. I didn't have to face my treatments feeling powerless and overwhelmed. I had tips and techniques to work with my body so it could process what was happening to it without succumbing to fear and pain. I thought to myself: How many people could be helped if I share these simple tools that are helping me through my treatments? And so, this book took root that day.

A Meridian Runs Through It

Throughout my treatment, I stayed at either Kimberly or Nathalie's house, depending upon their schedule and my needs. For this round, I was staying with Nurse Nathalie. She informed me that Days Three through Five post-chemo are typically the worst for side effects. That was definitely proving to be the case. My poor stomach was really bearing the brunt of the assault this time. I felt queasy to the point of vomiting. Nothing was moving through my system, and I could only lie down and rest. Food consisted of ginger tea and white rice. According to TCM, stomach meridian is always involved in breast cancer because it runs right through the breasts. In addition, worry is the emotion associated with stomach meridian so I was acutely aware that an imbalance in my stomach meridian energy was at the heart of my issue, but trying to resolve the underlying issues that facilitated my cancer was like trying to change a flat tire while driving down the highway at 70 miles per hour!

My painful mouth sores were back in full bloom. I woke up at 2 AM because of the pain and couldn't go back to sleep. My ever-present nausea was gnawing at me, and I didn't have the energy to do anything but lie there. I decided I could at least hold some *Radiant Circuits* points. I felt better for doing so, but the underlying nausea remained. I had no choice but to hunker down and ride out the storm till morning.

Holding Radiant Circuit Points

To activate Yin Regulator:

1. Place your right hand on the right side of your forehead in line with your right eye and your left hand somewhere along the inside of your left leg.
2. Hold these places for at least three to five minutes.
3. Switch sides and place your left hand on the left side of your forehead in line with your left eye and your right hand along the inside of your right leg.
4. Hold these places for at least three to five minutes.

NOTE: This technique is taught in greater detail on Pages 115-120.

The next day proved challenging because I had the worst bout of diarrhea since Day Three of Round 1. Becoming dehydrated might not sound like much, but it makes one weak and dizzy. I muddled through another day just trying to muster the energy to walk across the room. I didn't want to take more than one drug because I didn't want to stir up my skin allergy, which was finally dying down, but I had to break down and take Lomotil, a prescription medication for diarrhea. It worked, but by the end of the day, I was itching all over.

Quicksand

By Day Five, this disease was getting the best of me. After being beaten down by the side effects, I started to doubt myself. The message was loud and clear: Getting this disease made me a failure and a fraud. I failed on several counts, I surmised. Even though I am an EEM practitioner, I couldn't heal myself; therefore, I was a fraud. Even though I worked so hard to prove myself a success, I failed to do so. Once this mindset took hold, the negative thoughts started to go deeper. I was a failure because I couldn't figure out what I was supposed to do with my life until I was in my fifties. I didn't listen to my inner voice and insisted on resisting choices that I knew were in my best interest. When I finally figured out what I wanted to do with my life, I still failed!

By now, I was descending into the Realm of Regrets: What shoulda/coulda/woulda I done differently? In my zombie stupor state, I was remembering all the failures of my life: decisions I made that I regretted; failing my daughter; failing a friend who trusted me; betraying my parents; failing myself by not making the right choices. The regrets then led to self-doubt and, finally, a lack of self-worth - having to justify why I am here. Was that at the root of my disease? I don't deserve to live so I have an unconscious "death wish"?

By now, I was grasping at straws. How could I pull myself out of this muck? Part of me knew I was only hurting myself, yet I was down so deep in the mud, I couldn't move. Fortunately, **EFT** empowered me to extricate myself from this morass. It allowed me to reframe the issue and pull myself out of the quagmire. I started tapping while reciting these affirmations:

> *Even though I made mistakes, I'm still worthy of living.*
> *Even though I made mistakes, I don't deserve to die.*
> *Even though I made mistakes, some of those mistakes were beyond my control.*
> *Even though I made mistakes, I made the best choices I could at the time with the information that I had.*
> *Even though it took me years to figure out what I wanted to do with my life, I made the shifts to make it happen.*
> *Even though I started late, I built a successful practice from the ground up.*
> *Even though I am sick now, I helped thousands of people with the tools of energy medicine.*
> *Even though I have cancer, I helped many people with cancer get through their treatments successfully.*
> *Even though I am sick now, I have the tools of energy medicine to help me through this treatment.*

Within a few minutes, I pulled myself out of the victim mentality and mustered the energy to soldier onward.

The Emotional Freedom Technique

1. Decide what issue you want to work on. Work on only one issue at a time. This technique focuses on the negative emotion, so choose something that is actually bothering you.

2. Rate this issue on a scale of 0–10, 10 being the most triggering. If something is an actual 10, don't start with that issue. Choose something that is in the 7–8 range.

3. Even though you are working with a negative memory or issue, you want to choose an overall positive statement to tap into the acupuncture points. You will be making this statement out loud throughout this practice.

4. To begin the technique, bring the edges of your palms together—like a karate chop—while making this statement out loud:
   Even though I am struggling with _____, I love and accept myself as I am.

5. Make this statement three times while tapping the sides of your hands together.

6. Continue to tap on the following the points while making the statement out loud:
   a. Top of the head
   b. At both temples
   c. Under the eyes
   d. On top of the lip
   e. On the chin
   f. Under the collarbone
   g. On both sides of the ribcage
   h. On both sides of the legs

7. You can shorten the phrase while you tap through the body to something like:
   It's 7 on a scale of 0 -10 or *This _____ issue of mine.*

8. Tapping these points while making the statement constitutes one round of EFT.

9. Check in with yourself after each round to see if the original number has lowered.

10. Your goal is to get the number down to a 1 or 2.

   NOTE: This technique is described in greater detail on Page 186.

Calling in Reinforcements

As I continued to get more chemo, I became concerned that my body would build up too much toxicity, which would then become a problem. My liver and kidneys needed attention to process the medications I was receiving. Of course, I had my energy tools, but I wanted some alternative practitioners who could support me in my journey. As luck would have it, my health insurance policy had an accelerated death benefit option that paid me $15,000 because of my life-threatening illness. (Now that's a weird sensation—collecting your death benefit before you die!) I decided to use this money to help pay for the 30 different modalities I would explore during my treatment.

I found a well-respected local doctor known for using supplements and IV vitamin C therapy for his cancer patients, but he was booked three months out. I was almost halfway through my chemo treatment and couldn't wait three months. I had better luck connecting with Tom Tam and the Tong Ren Collective Healing Center. Tom is famous in the Boston area for helping cancer patients who are sent home to die. I knew about Tom from my work with cancer clients and had admired his approach; little did I know I'd be needing his help one day!

Tom Tam's healing system[7] combines a unique twist on the ancient techniques of Tuina massage and acupuncture to release blockages along the spinal column and allow blood, chi, bioelectricity and oxygen to feed a diseased organ. Tom also developed something called Tong Ren Healing which uses quantum physics to affect change in the body by means of an effigy.

I decided to attend one of Tom's Tong Ren healing classes. I was impressed by his demeanor and his passion for the work. He was humble and compassionate with a self-depreciating sense of humor. TCM teaches that human beings are a microcosm of nature's five elements: water, wood, fire, earth, and metal. Each of us has a predominant element that colors our personality and reveals our strengths and weaknesses. The goal of life is to become an equal expression of all five elements. Tom Tam is one of the few people I've ever met who appears to have achieved this balance.

華陀夾脊新註
TOM TAM HEALING SYSTEM

C1	Top of Head	頸1	頭頂
C2	Forehead	頸2	前額
C3	Eye, Sinus, Ear	頸3	眼、鼻、耳
C4	Mouth, Cheek, Chin	頸4	口、頰、頦
C5	Larynx, Pharynx	頸5	咽、喉
C6	Thyroid Gland	頸6	甲狀腺
C7	Parathyroid Glands	頸7	副甲狀腺
T1	Windpipe, Bone Marrow	胸1	氣管、骨髓
T2	Bronchus, Thymus Gland	胸2	支氣管、胸腺
T3	Lung, Lymph	胸3	肺、淋巴
T4	Breast, Sweat Gland, Hair Follicle	胸4	乳、汗腺、毛囊
T5	Heart (L) Pericardium (R)	胸5	心(左)、心包(右)
T6	Diaphragm	胸6	橫隔膜
T7	Spleen (L) Abdominal Blood Vessel (R)	胸7	脾(左)、腹腔管(右)
T8	Esophagus (L) Pancreas (R)	胸8	食道(左)、胰臟(右)
T9	Stomach (L) Liver (R)	胸9	胃(左)、肝臟(右)
T10	Gall Bladder (L) Bile Duct (R)	胸10	膽囊(左)、膽管(右)
T11	Small Intestine	胸11	小腸
T12	Transverse Colon	胸12	橫結腸
L1	Adrenal Gland, Testis, Vagina	腰1	腎上腺、睪丸、陰道
L2	Kidney, Seminal Vesicle, Uterus	腰2	腎、精囊、子宮
L3	Prostate, Ovary	腰3	前列腺、卵巢
L4	Large Intestine	腰4	大腸
L5	Descending Colon	腰5	降結腸
S1	Ureter	骶1	輸尿管
S2	Urinary Bladder	骶2	膀胱
S3	External Genital	骶3	外生殖器官
S4	Urinary Tract	骶4	尿道
S5	Rectum	骶5	直腸

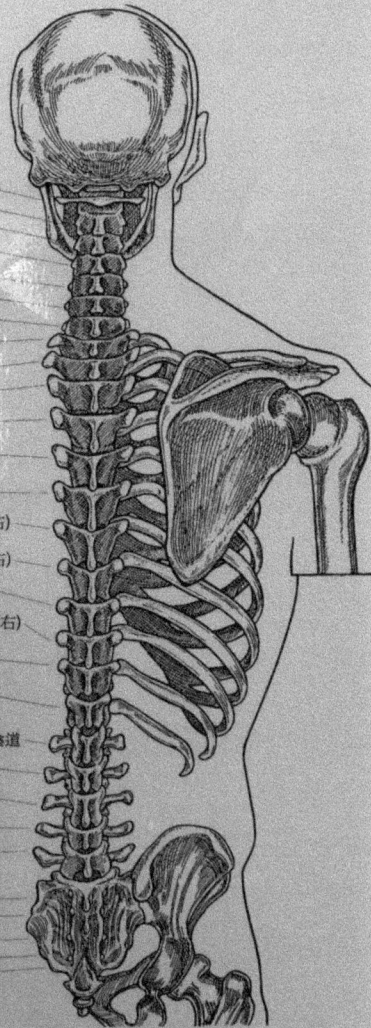

Oriental Culture Institute
東方文化學院

After I told Tom my diagnosis, he immediately made the connection between my underlying autoimmune issues and the inflammatory aspects of my cancer. I was surprised at how much he knew about IBC, making a correlation between something in my blood, the cancer, and my bone marrow not functioning well. That was surprising yet logical because in TCM, earth element governs the blood. In the human body, the earth element is comprised of the stomach and spleen meridians, which are always involved with breast cancer. I felt reassured that I had found someone who understood the underlying core issues that caused my cancer in the first place.

Tom told me that he had very good success healing IBC and I didn't have anything to worry about. That was reassuring to hear, of course, but I wasn't going to put all my eggs into the Tong Ren basket. Nevertheless, encountering Tom Tam, Tuina massage and Tong Ren Healing proved to be a pivotal part of my healing journey.

A Terrifying Prospect

About a week into Round Two, I was scheduled for a needle-guided biopsy on my left breast. My July mammogram showed some calcification in that breast and apparently, calcification can be a precursor to cancer. It was important to know this information because it would determine whether I would be getting a single or a double mastectomy.

Previously, I had prepared my body days in advance for what was about to transpire, but, somehow, I forgot this time. I almost had a panic attack because I remembered the agony of my first biopsy. I knew a needle biopsy would be painful and difficult. Fortunately, they couldn't get access to the calcification because it was in an awkward position, so they decided to do the biopsy at the time of my mastectomy. I would simply have to live with the uncertainty of knowing whether I would be undergoing a double or single mastectomy.

I also saw my oncologist that day and reported that I was having blurry vision. I suspected it was from one of the meds I was prescribed and thought she might adjust them, but she immediately suspected that my cancer had spread to my brain and ordered a PET scan. In addition, she reminded me that the radiology team in Washington, DC, reported seeing something abnormal on my pelvic CT scan, so she ordered a pelvic MRI, too. Apparently, I could be living with not just IBC, but also double breast, cervical, and even brain cancer!

My birthday was a few days later. Although I was surrounded by loved ones, I didn't feel much like celebrating; I was just going through the motions. Would I live to see another birthday? How would I be next year at this time? I was profoundly grateful for all that I had and all that I'd achieved in my life, but I was not ready to go yet. There was so much yet to accomplish and so much to live for.

The Fire It Burns

A couple of weeks post-chemo and my rash took on a life of its own. It was expanding and no one seemed to know what was causing it. Was it the chemo, the anti-diarrhea drug, or another medication? I had to avoid the sun at all costs because that made it worse.

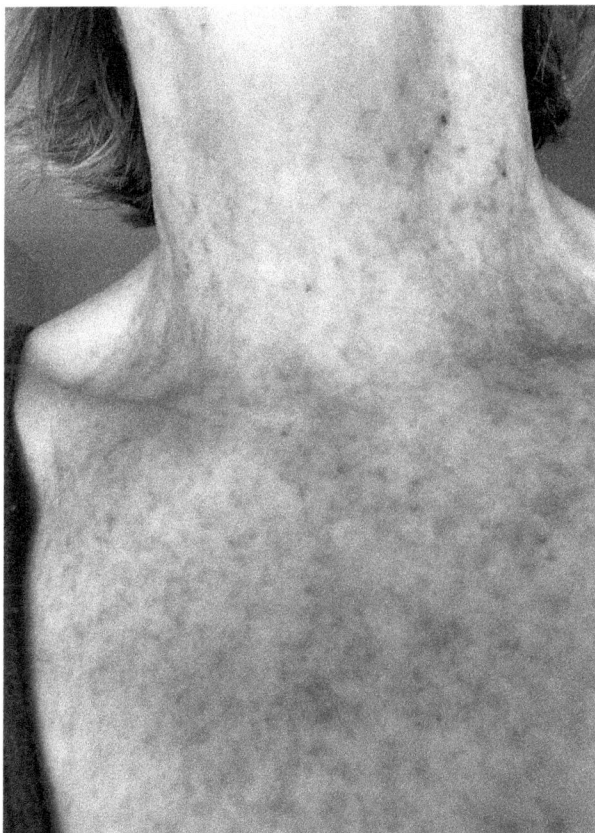

I used the hydrocortisone cream the doctor prescribed; the pain and itching got better where I applied it, but new lesions popped up almost immediately on other parts of my body.

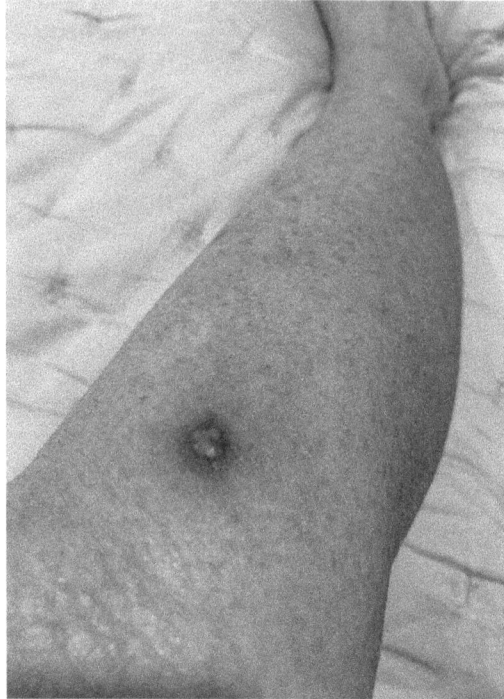

Exercising My Options

Having taught cancer patients and their families how to support themselves with energy medicine, I know it's ideal to have someone doing energy work on a daily basis as you undergo your treatment if possible. Unfortunately, even though Kim was an EEM practitioner, it wasn't always possible for her to work on me, so I decided to start doing qigong. I didn't have the strength to walk far, but I knew I needed to move my body. Like yoga, qigong works with the body's internal organs and circulates chi throughout the body. Because its movements are slow, qigong taps into the body's parasympathetic nervous system: the body's "rest and digest" response. After just one session, I was pleasantly surprised. I felt the benefits almost immediately, and they continued over the next several days. It is easy to do and almost effortless. Starting was as simple as finding a YouTube video that consisted of two ten-minute sessions, one in the morning and one in the evening.[8]

What's Around the Corner

As I started taking steroids to prepare for Round Three, I was feeling anxious because I didn't have the kind of support I wanted to have in place and I was already halfway through my chemo regime. My body was showing signs of toxicity: my eyesight was off, and my hair was falling out in gobs. I noticed signs of edema in my legs, and my rash had spread to my extremities. I cried off and on most of the day, not knowing whether it was from feeling sorry for myself or from fear of the unknown. It was the last day I had my body to myself before the next round and I was already exhausted. However, I did learn one thing about nature's design genius: Nose hairs are important. Without them, you become a blubbering mess when you cry!

I dreaded going on steroids because they completely changed my personality and prevented me from sleeping or eating. Just a few days before beginning the next round of chemo, I felt very apprehensive, sad, and overwhelmed. Kim's children were sick, so I was staying with Nurse Nathalie. While lamenting the onslaught of chemicals coming my way the next day, Nathalie said, "Mom, you know the power of the mind. Just tell your mind to rule over your body." I countered her dismissively saying, "Mind power is all well and good until your body is having toxins injected into it." I didn't give it a second thought until I realized that I was not going to get any outside help for the upcoming third round. Before Round Two, Kim balanced my energy systems, Heather, my therapist/friend, helped prepare my *triple warmer* (See Page 97) for the infusion, and Peggy, my massage therapist, prepared my body with Tuina massage.

Nathalie's prodding made me think: Yes, I was powerless to prevent the oncoming chemical onslaught, but I still had the power to change my attitude about it. I decided I needed to face my fear and figure out a way to shift my mindset. What tools did I have at my disposal? I needed something that was fast and simple because time was of the essence. It dawned on me that a combination of temporal tapping and EFT tapping might do the trick.

Using EFT, I was able to downregulate my anxiety and grief from an 8 to a 4. Tapping on acupuncture points, I said:

Even though I am very anxious about tomorrow's treatment, I deeply love and accept myself.
Even though my anxiety is at an 8, I am worthy of love and acceptance.
After several rounds of tapping on anxiety, this led to a bubbling up of grief:

Even though I feel sad and overwhelmed about what is to come, I still love and accept myself.
Even though my body is taking a hit, I am worthy of love and acceptance.

I continued to diffuse these emotions until the thoughts were no longer triggering.

Next, using temporal tapping, I decided to attack my body's reaction to the chemo head on—literally. I immediately started tapping on the following statements along the triple warmer meridian:

These drugs are going to kill off my cancer cells.
I'm not afraid of these cancer drugs.

I was starting to feel better. Plus, as depressed as I was that my drug regime was starting again, I forgot one positive thing about steroids: They give you so much energy! For the past three weeks, I could barely drag my body anywhere and doing a small task was an enormous undertaking. But after taking the steroids, I was able to go food shopping in a big grocery store, make dinner, organize my daughter's kitchen, and clean up afterwards without having to take a break. Plus, my appetite was ferocious! It was as if my body wanted to devour all the food that it wouldn't be able to enjoy over the next few weeks. Too bad steroids are bad for the bones: I could get used to this!

Chapter 4

The Poisoning

Making Lemonade

Everything I wrote about my infatuation with steroids during Round Two? Scratch that. I forgot about the heartburn that creeps in, the restless nights, and the racing thoughts that qigong, magnesium, ashwagandha, and melatonin couldn't manage to shut down. After not sleeping an entire night, I had to take a double dose of steroids. Perhaps it was the combination of steroids and the hydrocortisone I was putting on my chest, but I felt like I was going to jump out of my skin. Not the best of circumstances to start my day at the hospital.

Fortunately, when I couldn't sleep, I could always do energy medicine. Simple things that were literally at my fingertips because I can't reach too far or move too much. They included the following:

- *Opening the gaits.*
- Massaging *source points.* (See Page 169)
- Holding *meridian beginning and endpoints.* (See Page 139)
- Calming *triple warmer* meridian. (See Page 97)

Opening the Gaits

1. Open your right palm and with your left thumb, massage from the base of the right hand across the palm to each finger.
2. Moving to the little finger, continue to massage up the finger until you get to the tip.
3. Pull the energy off the little finger.
4. Move back to the base of the palm. Massage up the ring finger.
5. Take the energy off the ring finger.
6. Continue to do this with the rest of the fingers.
7. Turn the hand over and massage from the base of the hand at the wrist and move up to each finger.
8. Pull the energy off each fingertip.
9. Switch and do the left hand.

NOTE: A more detailed explanation of this technique can be found on Page 128.

So, even though I was pumped full of steroids and hadn't slept much, the combination of my temporal tapping and doing energy medicine on myself throughout the night lessened my feelings of stress and apprehension going into Round Three.

I met with a nurse practitioner this time. Thinking it would calm down the angry rash that had spread throughout my body, she decided to withhold the Perjeta, one of the chemo drugs I'd been receiving. Anytime a drug can be withheld, I consider that a win. I told her about my reactions to steroids, and she said I could cut them in half, too, or even eliminate them entirely in the future. (Oddly enough, whenever I asked a medical professional why they administer steroids during chemo, I'd get a different answer: Some said it was for nausea, while others said they simply didn't know why.)

When I was first diagnosed, I created a CaringBridge[9] web page to keep my friends, colleagues, students, clients, and family informed of my progress. So many people sent healing energy and prayed for me that, going into Round Three, I felt like I was being carried on calming waves of love and support. Despite my fears prior to beginning Round Three, it turned out to be the easiest so far!

Strategic Maneuvers

After feeling like I was behind the eight ball for several months, I finally lined up my support strategy. Initially, my overall cancer treatment plan was to throw everything at it including the kitchen sink, but after conducting countless hours of research and reading dozens of books, I decided to take a multipronged approach to my treatment consisting of the following:

- Tradition Western Medicine (chemo, surgery, and radiation)
- EEM and EFT
- Tom Tam's Tong Ren healing, acupuncture, and Tuina massage
- A metabolic approach that included supplements, exercise, and nutritional changes

It was my hope and intention that the combination of these tools would help me not just kill the cancer cells, but address the underlying terrain that allowed my disease to take root initially.

Thinking Outside the Box

During Round Three, I rediscovered PubMed[10]. PubMed is a NIH website that gives the public access to all of its published clinical studies. Twenty years ago, I used PubMed in the wee hours of the morning when I was searching for a stem cell transplant for Jonathan. It was a lifesaver then, and it would prove to be a huge help again. Whatever side effect I was struggling with, I could search this database for any relevant studies.

For example, I discovered a NIH study proving that kiefer, a milk-based product, can control chemo-induced diarrhea. Although I was excited to make this discovery, it surprised me that no one I encountered in the medical profession knew anything about this study. Many patients would prefer natural methods to address their side effects. Here was a clinical study proving that a natural product can alleviate medication-induced suffering, yet 90% of oncologists or oncology nurses most likely don't know about it. Why are these study results not filtering down to traditional hospitals so they can become standard of care?

This failure puts the burden on sick patients or their loved ones to do their own research. Many do, but most patients will simply defer to their doctors, regardless of whether the doctors have educated themselves on a particular alternative treatment. It is a disservice to advise patients not to do something just because doctors don't know the answer. For example, I had months of excruciating pain because my rash had spread throughout my body. I was desperate for relief from the constant pain and itching. I asked my oncologist about the possibility of using vitamin E on my skin, and she said, "I know nothing about vitamin E." At least she was honest!

The Roller Coaster Resumes

Despite my easy infusion experience, within a few days, I was transported back to Zombieland. I know now what they mean when they say the chemo's effects are cumulative. What began as indigestion and a lack of appetite led to vomiting. The rash I thought might be going away mushroomed on my back like never before. Not only was it ugly, it also generated large pustules that were so painful, I felt like I was being tortured day and night. This rash was in the running for being the worst side effect of all.

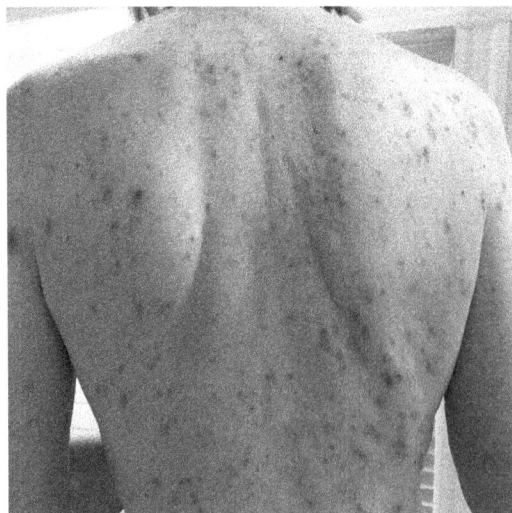

Chapter 5

The Poisoning

Round Four: October 1, 2021

The Ugly Elephant in the Room

Yep, my rash *was* becoming my worst side effect. It was intensifying and slowly creeping up my neck and extremities, and it was oozing and raw. I was in constant pain and couldn't sleep. I resorted to taking long baking soda baths and drenching my skin in calamine lotion hoping to get a short respite from the constant itching. It would help for about 20 minutes, but then the painful itching would come roaring back.

For some reason, no one wanted to say it was chemo-induced skin lupus. The nurse practitioner insisted the rash was from the massages I was getting, not the Perjeta. She wanted to reintroduce the Perjeta, but I was adamant. I could not take that drug. Whenever I took it, I couldn't move my head off the bed for a week. I was told I couldn't be seen by a dermatologist for six months. She recommended seeing an oncology dermatologist the following week. Now I had to worry about skin cancer, too?

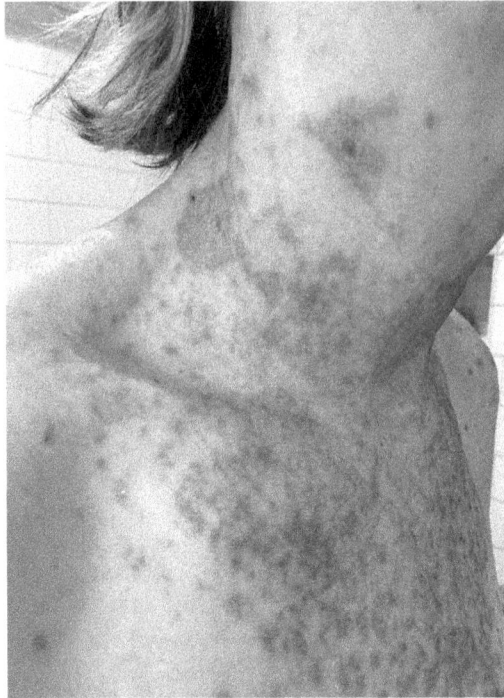

I decided instead to see an allergist who declared that my rash was environmentally created, not chemo-induced. He did a battery of allergy tests, which all came back negative. (This was interesting because prior to doing EEM, I was allergic to nearly all grasses and trees.) The ointment he prescribed burned my skin and made the rash worse. By this point, I was wondering: Which drug is causing this? Will my skin look like this for the rest of my life?

Zombie Apocalypse

Two weeks later, I should have been feeling better, but I wasn't. So far, Round Four had been the hardest to bounce back from. In addition to the regular cast of characters—stomach queasiness, no appetite, mouth sores, a lack of energy, and diarrhea—neuropathy and bone pain arrived. I might have had an inkling of these issues in prior rounds, but, this time, it was as if someone turned up the volume button to full blast and it was not going back down. I could barely breathe. Everything hurt: my ribcage, my shoulders, even my jaw; the pain would move around my body. It felt as though my bones were having the life sucked out of them while simultaneously, somebody was sitting on top of me and crushing me. I could only walk with the help of walking sticks. I had to find a way to deal with these side effects without having to take more drugs!

Stuck Inside the Box

When I called my oncologist's office to report the bone pain, all she could offer me was oxycodone. More drugs, and addictive ones at that. With some research, Nurse Nathalie discovered that over-the-counter allergy medicines like Claritin could help with bone pain. She also learned that sucking on ice chips while getting chemo can prevent mouth sores. Later, when I asked my infusion nurse for a cup of ice chips, she giggled and said, "Oh, that's a patient thing." Really? Is it just a "patient thing"?

Checking online, I found that most cancer sites state something similar: "Some *patients* (italics added) find sucking on ice chips helps." Nothing from the medical community confirms this approach. However, a NIH study demonstrated that sucking on ice chips can prevent mouth sores. For some reason, this information is not filtering down to the medical institutions that are treating cancer patients. A 2017 study in the *Journal of the National Cancer Institute* reported that wearing ice packs on the hands or feet for 90 minutes after a chemo infusion can help prevent neuropathy. Despite already having four rounds of chemotherapy, I was never offered ice packs.

Discovering the cure to my chronic chemo-induced diarrhea happened by sheer accident. During a visit with her nutritionist, Kim mentioned I was having chemo-induced diarrhea, and the nutritionist recommended calcium bentonite clay. Although kiefer had been helping to keep my digestive system calm, the calcium bentonite clay was an actual cure. When I queried my oncology nutritionist if she'd ever heard of it, she hadn't.

Curious to see whether there were any studies conducted on calcium bentonite clay, sure enough, I found several in PubMed. Multiple studies have shown the many benefits of using bentonite clay to detoxify the body. So, after suffering four rounds of chemo, I finally found relief from some of the worst chemo side effects without prescription drugs and by using simple, natural methods that have studies to back them up. Yet virtually no one in oncology knows about them? I find that both odd and disturbing.

Shining a Light

When in the throes of cancer treatment, it's difficult to see the light at the end of the tunnel. Often, it feels as though you've lost yourself and your body, and you don't know if you will ever feel like yourself again. It's a kind of limbo state where you are just existing, waiting to be liberated. I remember when Jon was being treated, I said to his doctors, "You need to have some kind of Hall of Hope with photos of survivors who got through their treatment and are doing well so patients undergoing treatment will have the strength to carry on, knowing they can get through the trauma."

Learning from survivors is critical towards that end, but for some reason, I was unable to connect with an IBC survivor until four months into my treatment. This absence of support left me in a state of confusion and fear. I wanted to be certain that I had no option but to have both surgery and radiation after chemo. Moreover, I wanted to know if there was anyone who survived treatment and was living a normal life without suffering long-term side effects.

The first survivor I spoke with was 12 years post-treatment and had no late effects. Unfortunately, however, her mother, who also had IBC, chose not to undergo radiation after having surgery and died within five months. The second woman I spoke with was four years post-treatment, but she still suffered from chronic issues of neuropathy and gastroparesis, a paralysis of the stomach caused by nerve damage. Both of these conditions were incurable for her. She was philosophical about her late effects, saying, "It's the price you pay to stay alive."

My End Game

Although energy work, acupuncture, and massage helped me manage my cancer treatment, everything ramped up during Round Four so I was not in great shape facing Round Five in a few days. A friend gave me a beautiful green stone that read: *Believe in Miracles*. I wondered: What would a miracle look like for me? I had witnessed miracles with Jon's cancer story, but at 65, I started this journey with a lifetime of stress, underlying medical risk factors, and wear and tear on my body. To walk this path and emerge on the other side cancer-free, without incurring any debilitating late effects that need medication would be ideal. From what I'd seen thus far, that would be a miracle!

Chapter 6

The Poisoning

Round Five: October 22, 2021

Crunch Time

I met with the oncologist for the first time in two rounds and learned that, because of the IBC's aggressiveness, a radical mastectomy must be performed within three to four weeks of finishing chemo. Radiation should begin four weeks post-surgery. Because of my rash, side effects, and concern for late effects, we discussed the possibility of skipping Round Six and going right into surgery. However, the extent to which residual cancer might remain in the tumor can be known only at the time of surgery, and the answer to that question impacts one's prognosis.

Consequently, I was faced with the Damoclean dilemma of deciding whether the risk of forgoing Round Six would outweigh the benefit of preventing more long-term side effects. The good news was the doctor didn't add back the Perjeta and she cut my chemo by 20%. She also lowered my steroid dose and agreed to give it to me by IV.

Despite the fact that this was Round 5, I handled it the best so far. I even had the strength to do my daily energy exercises.

Staying Grounded on a Daily Basis

1. Place your middle finger into your navel.
2. Place your other middle finger at the middle of your forehead.
3. Push in on both fingers and pull upwards as if you are creating a line from your navel to your third eye (middle forehead).
4. Breathe in slowly through your nose and out through your mouth.
5. Hold this position for a minute or two.

NOTE: This technique is explained more fully on Page 195.

The bentonite clay stopped the diarrhea in its tracks. Sucking on ice chips prevented me from developing mouth sores, and taking Claritin nipped the bone pain in the bud. I was tired and slept long hours, but I wasn't comatose like before. Cutting the chemo dosage by 20% seemed to have helped too. Despite these advantages, however, my skin rash continued to rage on.

Oddly enough, the agonizing sores covered my entire body with the exception of my right breast, where the cancer lived.

It was finally sinking in that I was going to have major surgery in the not-too-distant future. A daunting prospect—losing one's breast and considering what life would be like on the other side. I apologized to the breast and thanked her for her service. I did lots of EFT tapping to work through the emotions associated with the loss and made my peace with it. I'm not sure I would have been so quick to achieve that peace of mind if I had been 20 or 30 years younger.

I also met my radiology oncologist. I had heard good things about him, but he outperformed his stellar reputation. As fearful as I was about the prospect of radiation, meeting him was one of the best experiences I'd had so far. After seeing my rash, he immediately referred me to a dermatologist. He also said he would collaborate with me on the amount of radiation I might receive. Despite his help, it would be another month before I finally would see a dermatologist.

Chapter 7

The Poisoning

Round Six: November 11, 2021

That's a Wrap

November 11th was supposed to be my last round of chemo, but my blood counts were so low, they couldn't administer it. If the counts had been just a few points lower, I would have needed a transfusion. Phew—I dodged that bullet! I did have a Herceptin infusion, but I was officially done with chemo. I felt a little vulnerable, however, because with IBC, surgery is supposed to be within three to four weeks of the last chemo treatment, which would no longer be the case for me. Now I had a choice: Wait for my blood counts to come up and have another round of chemo or have surgery in a week. Since surgery is the supposed cure, why postpone the inevitable? Why put more poison into my body? I decided to take my chances and schedule the surgery.

The Human Pin Cushion

Having major surgery is not as simple as booking it and showing up on that day. There are lots of preparatory twists and turns that involve things like having radioactive seeds placed into one's body. In my case, the bullet I dodged with a scheduled biopsy a few months ago was coming back to haunt me. Before going under the knife, I needed to have a needle-guided mammogram to determine the exact location of the calcification in my left breast. A radioactive "seed" would be placed to guide the surgeon during the biopsy. I'd never had a needle-guided mammogram, but I've had the biopsy/mammogram from hell, and this sounded like one of those!

First came a regular mammogram to locate the area of calcification. Next, lidocaine was injected to numb the breast. Then a five-inch needle was inserted into the side of the breast. The needle stayed in there while numerous photos were taken from various angles— all while my breast was being compressed in the mammogram machine. This went on for close to an hour. I would have been okay, but they asked me to keep standing while they compressed the breast with the needle sticking out on the side. At some point, I was so nauseated, I had to lay down; the tears started to flow.

Hello, Darkness, My Old Friend

With my surgery just a week away and feeling traumatized from my needle-guided mammogram, I was agitated, anxious, and unable to relax. I hadn't felt this way in many years and wondered if my triple warmer had moved into reactivity mode. ***Triple warmer reactivity*** (See Page 98) is the Eden Method's term for post-traumatic stress disorder (PTSD). Under prolonged stress or trauma, the brain's limbic system can't shift from sympathetic into parasympathetic response and effectively gets stuck in a reactive stress response loop. Once triple warmer reactivity gets a toe hold, it's difficult to reverse. I lived most of my life in triple warmer reactivity, never knowing it wasn't "normal," but energy medicine taught me how to reverse that condition. Apparently, my needle-guided mammogram was a new trauma that triggered the old trauma of my first biopsy, and my body moved into stress reactivity. Doing the ***triple warmer reactivity pose*** helped, but it wasn't until Kim held my ***neurovascular points*** and cleared my chakras that my body finally calmed down and I felt at peace.

Holding the Main Neurovasculars

1. Place one palm of your hand on your forehead and the other behind the back of your head directly behind your eyes. Be sure that your hands are *lightly* touching your head. You don't want to compress your hands on the head or it will block the flow of blood, oxygen, and energy.
2. Breathe in through your nose and out through your mouth. Try to hold the pose for at least three to five minutes or until you find your body releasing its stress response.

NOTE: This technique is explained in greater detail on Page 97.

Death by a Thousand Cuts

My scheduled surgery was continually postponed because my blood counts were still too low. As they say, "Chemo is the gift that keeps on giving." Even though I hadn't had any since October 22nd, it was still in my system, and I was experiencing its cumulative side effects. I was extremely fatigued. I had a sore throat, and there was a strange stye in my eye that wouldn't heal. And beyond all those things, my skin nightmare had entered a new phase. The patches of painful lesions that were on my neck and chest had now crept up to my face, so I couldn't hide them. Scaly scabs that oozed and bled covered every part of my body. Just when I thought they couldn't get any worse, they did. Fortunately, I had an appointment with a dermatologist the next day, so I clung to hope that he would solve this riddle.

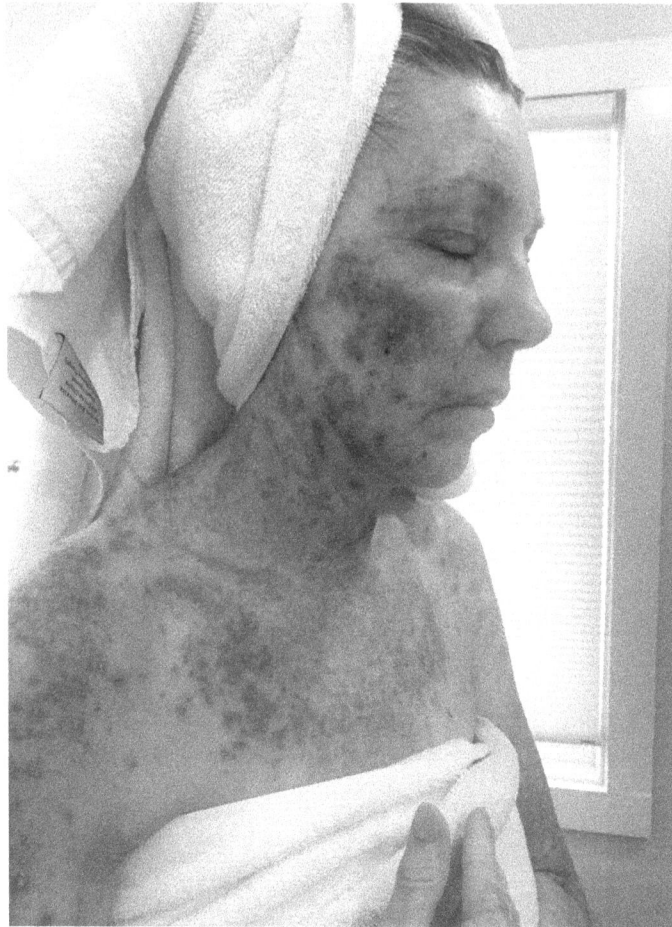

Never Looking Back

When I finally saw the dermatologist, he looked at me and said, "This looks like a chemo-therapy allergic reaction." His biopsies (two more biopsies!) confirmed what I already knew, but at least we found the actual culprit: Taxotere-induced skin lupus. I thought he would prescribe Plaquenil, a common lupus drug, but he said it would take months for it to work, and, by then, the chemo would have left my system. He prescribed betamethasone, an ointment to be used temporarily in small doses. Finally! Something to douse the fire. It worked for the pain, but could it heal the skin, or would I be scarred for life? Surgery was just days away: How would my skin react to it? Would the chemo leave my system before radiation began?

With my back against the wall, I decided I would do whatever it took to rid myself of this scourge. I might not be able to cure myself of cancer, but I knew there were things I could do to counteract skin lupus. EEM had cured me of my auto-immune issues years before, but that was before I had chemo injected into my body every three weeks. Scouring the internet late into the night, I came upon the story of a physician who cured her lupus by changing her diet. She wrote a book, *Goodbye Lupus[11]*, about her experience. Her diet was essentially vegan: no dairy, no gluten, no processed foods, no sugar, no meat. I decided to take the leap and follow her lead.

Fist Punched and Manhandled

My needle-guided mammogram showed an enlarged left axillary lymph node, which could be my body's reaction to the skin lupus, but cancer needed to be ruled out, so yet another biopsy! My white cells were still low which delayed surgery again. I had to meet with a hematologist to rule out that my low blood counts weren't due to a blood cancer. I lost track of how many potential cancers I stared down. My life consisted of driving an hour back and forth to Boston to be pricked, poked, punctured, and pummeled. By the end of this nightmare, Jean-Pierre and I would have driven more than 30,000 miles and I would have had more than 120 blood draws, infusions, injections, or procedures.

Trying to put a positive spin on this latest biopsy, I decided it was an "appetizer" of what was to come. I hadn't had major surgery for more than 20 years, so I decided that this procedure could prepare my body for the pain of surgery. Because I was being treated in a teaching hospital, residents are sometimes in the room with the doctor. This time, however, the resident was the one performing the procedure. It was clear he had never done anything like this before and I was his guinea pig. Fortunately, the attending doctor was excellent and guided him well. At the end of the procedure, however, he couldn't stop the bleeding, probably because of my low platelet count. Rather than using his palm to exert pressure, he used his fist. He pressed and pushed with all his might and when he was done, I had the imprint of each one of his knuckles under my arm.

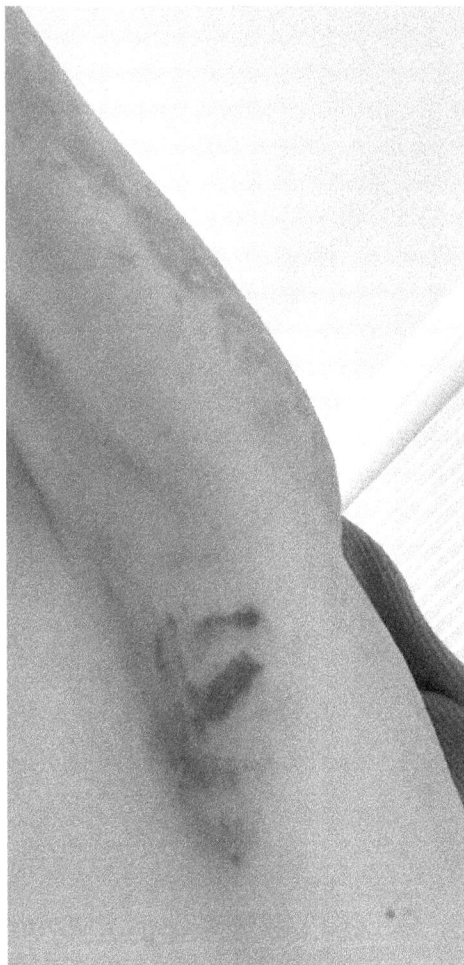

The Final Day

One day away from my mastectomy, I was keenly aware that this was the last day I would be the whole person I had been my entire life. On the following day, I would be disfigured and embarking on a trip with many pitfalls and potential dangers. I met my surgeon again and realized she was quite young. I checked her out on the hospital's website, and it was worse than I thought: She was only 32 years old! Having gone through medical school and residency, she could only have been in private practice for a couple of years at best. This really gave me pause.

Should I try to find someone older, someone with more experience? I struggled and prayed about this, but decided that the Universe gave me this surgeon for a reason and I needed to trust her capabilities.

Daily injections of Neupogen to counteract my neutropenia temporarily beefed up my white cells so I could get through surgery without the risk of infection. IBC requires a modified radical mastectomy, meaning the removal of the entire breast along with as much skin and as many lymph nodes as can be accessed. A biopsy of the left breast would also be performed during the surgery. Drains would be placed near the incision to taper off fluid buildup due to the lymph node removal.

I knew I would be grieving at some points, but for two days, I had lots of energy and was happy. I wanted and needed to hold onto that state of mind and use it to help my body accept this experience as a positive one instead of a negative one. I wanted my triple warmer to be happy that the root of the cancer that could have killed me would be taken out by the core, never to return. The breast itself felt dead, so it was only logical that the dead parts would be cut away. Temporal tapping and EFT would allow my body to accept this change.

Chapter 8

The Amputation

December 14, 2021

I said to my son-in-law the day before surgery, "I can't die because I don't know where my will is." So … I am still here. I survived! I might have even reconciled my disdain for hospitals. Not that I want to go there again anytime soon, but overall, my experience was good. The staff was pleasant and helpful—even the food was edible. I had a quiet room, so I was not disturbed by a lot of beeping or talking. I could turn the lights down, so the glare of fluorescent lights did not bother me. Those memories with Jonathan of spending countless nights in the hospital with the bright lights, constant beeping, and terrible food were abated, and my worst fears of going under the knife never materialized.

Post-Op Week One

I was told the surgery went well. The incision was about ten inches long, starting under my arm and going to the center of my torso. Two drains below the incision would remain in place for a week or two. The incision stitches were held together with purple glue, but I couldn't bring myself to look at them.

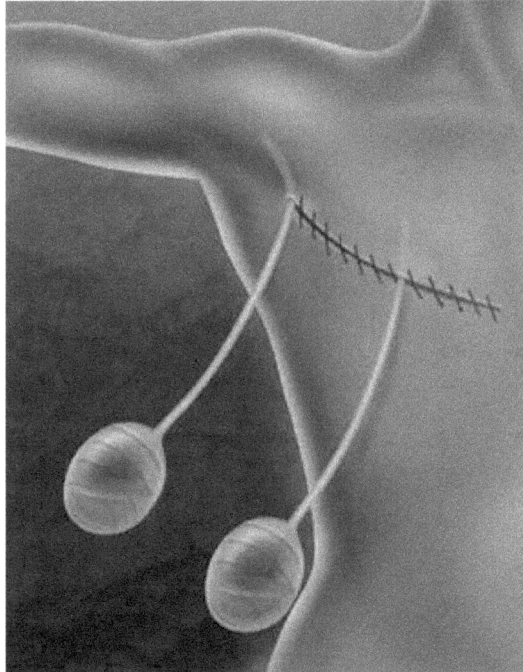

Nathalie rented a medical chair that allowed me to transition from sitting to standing by pushing a lever thereby putting no pressure on my arms. I would be sleeping in it for the next two weeks. I could walk around by myself unassisted. Although I couldn't do much but rest, overall, I was doing better than I expected. I was prescribed gabapentin and oxycodone for the pain and given daily exercises to increase my range of motion and help me regain muscle strength, but I couldn't raise my arm laterally more than a few inches.

Kim came over to do energy work on me. All my chakras were blown, and my biofield was nonexistent, but I was not homolateral or triple warmer reactive. That was remarkable!

How to Calm Triple Warmer Reactive Energies

1. Make an OK sign with your pointer and thumb.
2. Turn your hand and place the tip of your thumb and back of your pointer finger onto your temples.
3. Gently place the rest of your fingers across your forehead.
4. The baby finger should rest at the inside edges of your eyebrows. Your ring finger should be placed along the middle of the forehead and your middle finger should be touching your hairline.
5. Hold these positions lightly for at least three minutes or until you feel your stress response calming down.

NOTE: This technique is taught in greater detail on Page 98.

The pathology report would take two weeks and would bring with it the answers to these burning questions:

- How much of the tumor remains?
- What percentage is still cancerous?
- Are the cancer cells still HER2+?
- Were any lymph nodes involved?
- Are the margins around the tissue clear?
- What is the tumor's grade?
- Were there any hormone receptors present?

The answers to these questions would determine my ultimate prognosis.

I wanted to wean myself off the gabapentin because it was making my feet numb. I tried replacing it with oxycodone, but I immediately started itching, so I added oxycodone to my extensive list of drug allergies. The drains were becoming painful and annoying, so I resorted to calling them Thing 1 and Thing 2. Twice a day, I had to measure how much fluid they drained; they could be removed once the total was less than 30 milliliters a day. A visiting nurse was also giving me daily heparin injections to lower the risk of blood clots.

Besides the risk of the cancer returning, IBC patients also face the prospect of developing lymphedema because a significant amount of lymph nodes are removed during surgery. Lymphedema is a chronic, painful swelling of the arm caused by a compromised lymphatic system. A cut, infection, change in air pressure, or lifting too much weight can trigger it. Once it takes root, there is no cure; it can only be managed. Approximately 50% of all IBC survivors will develop it at some point in their lives.

I had seen clients with lymphedema in my practice, and I knew how difficult it is to treat. Having lymphedema would end my career. I learned my lesson of waiting too long to line up providers, so I lost no time in scheduling appointments with physical and occupational therapists to learn what I could do to prevent it. I also started the daily exercises I was given at the hospital to prevent developing frozen shoulder, another common side effect of a mastectomy.

Post-Op Week Two

I spent a day in Boston, going between two hospitals, one for a surgery follow-up and the other for my cancer treatment. I saw the oncologist first, who was surprised to see me in a wheelchair. I was surprised that she was surprised! One week out of major surgery with drains in? What was she thinking?

She announced she would not give me the Herceptin infusion because she thinks I still have cancer in my breast. She said she could feel the tumor bed and it could be filled with dead cells, but in her experience, if the bed remains, there tends to still be cancer cells there. If so, I would need to get targeted chemo along with Herceptin (a drug called Kadcyla) for the next year. This was very upsetting. Just when I thought I was at the finish line, the goal posts were moved. She also said it was not customary practice to receive heparin shots post-surgery, but because I was so fragile, they decided to administer it. I was not a happy camper by the end of that appointment!

I was finally able to have Thing 2 removed, but the next day, I woke up with what looked like an infection at the drainage site. It was about the size of a golf ball and was filled with fluid. My entire right flank was in pain. Worse than after the surgery itself. With Christmas just two days away, this was not on my Wish List.

No one told me, but apparently this can happen to people who undergo surgery. Ideally, Thing 1 would have drained into Thing 2, but that did not happen. Instead, my arm and underarm blew up; I could not move or raise my arm due to the excruciating pain. No one called or wrote back when I sent them photos, and I finally had to page the doctor after hours on Christmas Eve. We did not know if it was an infection, and Nurse Nathalie was thinking I might develop sepsis – a poisoning of the blood stream that can be fatal. Instead of visions of sugar plums dancing in my head, I suddenly had visions of spending Christmas in the hospital instead.

Fortunately, the doctor called back, looked at the photos, and proclaimed the golf-ball-size visitor a seroma—an accumulation of fluid from the surgery site that needed to be reabsorbed by the body. Nurse Nathalie applied warm compresses and significant pressure to encourage the fluid to flow back into the body cavity. Even though the doctor felt certain it was a seroma based on the photos, they still wanted to see me in the office the next day.

Interestingly, it had been just two days since my oncology appointment and I didn't need a wheelchair this time, so I was definitely regaining my strength. I saw a nurse practitioner who confirmed it was as seroma, not an infection and reassured me it was a common reaction to the surgery. She added that my scar and the skin around it looked great and I should be concerned only if I got chills or a fever.

At the end of the appointment, I asked her whether I could take arnica for the pain, explaining that it was an herbal remedy. When the nurse practitioner heard the word *herbal*, her entire countenance changed to one of fear. She said she knew nothing about arnica (it is sold in every drug store for pain) and, since there were no studies, I should not take it. Of course, I had to go home and check out PubMed. I did not find one study proving the effectiveness of arnica for pain: I found 69!

Almost two weeks out and my goal was to be off all pain meds within the week. I was diligently doing my strengthening exercises because, for radiation, I had to be able to raise my arm above my head every day for 30 days. The entire right side of my body was stiff, and the exercises didn't feel like they were making much of a dent. I had to keep doing them, though, or my entire right arm, shoulder and torso would freeze up. I asked my doctor how long into the future I would need to do them, and he replied, "For the rest of your life." My incision was painful and numb at the same time—a very weird sensation. I asked him when the numbness would go away, and he said, "Most likely never."

My seroma had a strange way of getting soft and then suddenly spasming and getting hard. I could also have been experiencing what was known as *chording*. Chording is a mysterious phenomenon that medical science cannot explain. It happens to some patients who have had multiple lymph nodes removed because either nerves were cut under the arm or because the lymph channels that were cut harden. It causes pain anytime you reach for something; it feels like there are guitar-like strings pulling inside your arm. It can last for weeks or forever. Fortunately, I had not experienced it yet; I was still trying to resolve the seroma. At times like these, it was handy to be a massage therapist because I could put my skills to practice moving the lymph, compressing the seroma, and pushing the fluid backwards to the source of the inflammation.

Post-Op Week Three

I found out the results of my left breast biopsy and right modified radical mastectomy:

Left Breast: No Evidence of Cancer
Right Breast Lymph Nodes: No Evidence of Cancer.
Sixteen had been removed. Two were necrotic, meaning the original stage lll diagnosis involved only two lymph nodes and those were killed with the chemo, so the cancer had not spread beyond those two nodes.
Residual cancer in tumor bed: 5%
Margins: Clear
HER2 Status: Negative
Hormone Receptor Status: Progesterone and Estrogen Positive

Breast cancers are classified into four hormone receptor categories: human epidermal growth factor (HER), progesterone, (PR), estrogen (ER) or no receptors (Triple Negative). Which of these categories your cancer falls into will determine what treatment you receive. Apparently, I changed from being HER2+ to HER2– and became progesterone and estrogen positive. This was highly unusual. Nurse Nathalie and I were baffled by this news. It meant either I had another kind of cancer prior to the IBC, or the hormone-positive cells were overpowered by the HER2+ cells in the original biopsy.

As we muddled our way through the report trying to decipher the meaning of *turbo*, *nuclear*, and *mitosis ratings*, she and I concluded that I had a Grade ll prognosis—not great with this cancer. Then we spoke with the nurse practitioner, who, after reviewing the report, said it was not good news, it was GREAT NEWS! She did not know much about the hormone receptor changes, but the fact that the cancer had responded so well to the chemo and had not spread—this was great news.

The seroma was still there, and the doctors were concerned that it might be getting infected, so there was a discussion that I might have to go on antibiotics. Since antibiotics and I do not get along well, I resolved to do whatever I could to prevent an infection. Something the visiting nurse said confirmed what I had been thinking. She explained that a post-surgery seroma is the body's way of filling up the space of what has just been removed. That made perfect sense. I just lost 16 lymph nodes, and my body had been trying to come back into balance from that loss. Now that was something I could deal with! I could have a conversation with my body and explain that it does not need to fill up that space. I could help it adjust to the changes with temporal tapping and EFT, telling my immune system that, as much as it has been trying to bring balance back to my body, it does not need to create the seroma. It does not need to fill up the space. I could give my body another message by tapping in:

> *My body knows how to drain its fluids beautifully.*
> *I do not need to fill in the lost space with a seroma.*

I tapped in this message about five times a day. Between that and the lymphatic drainage massage, I managed to avoid going on antibiotics.

There was significant pain under my arm, behind the armpit and down the back of my arm. I wanted to get off my prescription pain meds that week, but I could see this was not going to happen. I went for a walk, and by the end of it, my toes were numb, my incision hurt, and I felt overwhelmed. I took a shower and finally looked at the incision for the first time: I could not stop crying.

Whenever I have a health challenge, I try to educate myself as much as possible about the issue. I already knew a fair amount about the lymphatic system because it was a big focus of my EEM practice. The lymphatic system has more vessels than the circulatory system. The "garbage collector" of the body and an integral part of the immune system, its job is to filter toxins like viruses, bacteria, and dead cells from the body and regulate fluid in the tissues. Unlike the blood, which has a pump to filter it (the heart), the lymphatic system is stimulated only by movement, breathing, and massage.

Wanting to educate myself more about lymphedema in particular, I watched a YouTube video from a National Lymphedema Network symposium[12]. The speaker reported that medical doctors receive only 15 minutes of education on the lymphatic system in medical school. He then held up a large book on the lymphatic system and said, "Every doctor should know what is in this book because the lymphatic system is the body's immune system." That was an amazing statement: *The lymphatic system is the body's immune system, and doctors spend only 15 minutes learning about it?*

This really struck a nerve. I had worked in the medical field and treated those patients who were still grappling with the side effects of their various surgeries years later. The oncologist thinks, "I saved you from your cancer. My job is done." The surgeon thinks, "I saved you from your cancer. My job is done." The radiation oncologist thinks, "I minimized the risk of your cancer returning. My job is done." Physicians are not trained to think about the long-term side effects of chemo, surgery, and radiation. Clinical studies are not designed to take them into account. The fallout is relegated to the "lesser professions" of physical, occupational, and massage therapy. These practitioners and their patients are left to pick up the pieces.

Although it was New Year's Day I was in no mood to celebrate. Having digested the surgery and all that it entailed, I now had to turn my attention to the next chapter on my journey: radiation. In the past, I avoided excess radiation whenever possible. Now I would be spending weeks under its influence, with its many risks. The short-term side effects run the gamut of skin peeling, pain, burning, scarring, fatigue, adhesions, and esophageal and neck pain. Although the intention is to prevent the cancer from returning at the scar line, the radiation would be directed to not just that area, but to the entire right torso from the clavicle to the lateral lower rib cage and under the arm from the axillary to the base of the rib cage.

There are long-term effects of radiation as well: heart disease, radiation fibrosis, radiation pneumonitis, pulmonary fibrosis, cognitive decline, bone fractures, and an increased risk for lymphedema and secondary cancers. Many of these risks are compounded if one is receiving either chemotherapy or immunotherapy simultaneously. The scariest part is these side effects may not show up until years later.

Several people said to me, "Don't do the radiation. You are cured now; you do not need it." Or, "It will also kill healthy cells or create more damage. Once radiation kills cells, they can never be repaired." Of course, there was a part of me that would love to make that choice, but I happened to get the type of cancer for which that is not an option. So, reluctantly, I had to board the radiation train that would take me to a cancer-free life. In many ways, it could be the most difficult chapter in my recovery.

By now, I was supposed to see the oncologist and receive my next infusion. This would have included Kadcyla, a drug that combines Herceptin and T-DMI, a chemotherapy drug that was so deadly when administered alone it was taken off the market. Now, piggy-backed onto the immunotherapy agent Herceptin, it is considered to be the standard of care for HER2+ women who have any residual cancer post-mastectomy.

There are 45 common side effects from this medication, including nausea, fatigue, neuropathy, constipation, neutropenia (low white counts) and increased liver enzymes. The more serious side effects include liver damage, heart damage (dysfunction of the left ventricle), interstitial lung disease and thrombocytopenia (low platelet count). My oncologist claimed it is well-tolerated, but there is a Facebook group specifically dedicated to Kadcyla and its side effects. Read it and weep.

Post-Op Week Four

I was supposed to get Kadclya, but because I switched from being HER2+ to HER2−, I no longer fit the parameters for receiving it. I also still had low platelet and blood counts. This must be rare because the doctor said she would consult with the entire oncology team to get their feedback. In the interim, I would be getting Herceptin. She confirmed I was stage 1, which means I have the same prognosis as someone with a complete remission.

The oncologist was surprised to see that the pathology report showed I was now estrogen and progesterone positive since that hadn't shown up in the original biopsy. She said I would have to go on estrogen blockers right away. Typically, one is on hormone blockers between five and ten years. She wanted me to have a bone density test before starting because estrogen therapy has a risk of osteoporosis. But what is the point of that? If they put me on the drug and then I develop osteoporosis, then what? They would just put me on another drug. Not a good strategy for me. I have seen the side effects from estrogen blockers and osteoporosis drugs; ironically, they can destroy your bones. At my age, this would be an extremely risky proposition, so I chose to delay making that decision.

I was about to start physical therapy (PT) and wanted to get off the pain meds, so I decided to try a marijuana gummy to see if it would help with the pain. I ate half a gummy and felt nothing. About six hours later, I ate the second half. Then, I did feel something. My body relaxed, and the muscles that had been so stiff and painful turned into marshmallows. My brain turned into a marshmallow too. I went downstairs and ate two ice cream bars and some other things that I do not remember now because it was all a blur. I woke up the next day completely hung over. Marijuana gummies are a great solution if you are in pain, have no appetite, and do not need to function in the real world!

I came across one of my first journal entries from Round One of chemo, and I actually wrote, "I'm doing pretty well." At the six-month or "halfway'" mark from where I began, I can say that I have managed to survive and to my knowledge, I do not have severe life-threatening issues, but when I look at myself in the mirror, I do not recognize this stranger. My skin is dry and decrepit. I have the telltale butterfly red rash on my cheeks from lupus. My head has big holes in it where the hair has fallen out and the wisps of hair that are growing back are white or gray. My left hip hurts when I walk. My scar throbs by the end of the day, and my feet become numb if I walk too much.

I had an appointment for what was supposed to be my mapping for radiation, but I could not raise my arm up above my head. They looked at my scar, said it was too fresh and told me to come back in a week.

Post-Op Week Five

I had my second PT session today. I worked hard because I wanted to be able to hold my arms up for the radiation treatment, but everything was painful. A new extremely contagious variation of COVID-19 was going around, and Kim and Jean-Pierre came down with it. They were both quite sick, and Jean-Pierre was alone with no one to take care of him. Since I had just spent time with them both, Nurse Nathalie suggested I be tested. To my surprise, I tested positive. Other than a stuffy nose, I had no symptoms. I had to cancel my PT appointments, but I could not postpone the radiation. Therefore, I was now tasked with retraining my muscles alone so I would be able to undergo radiation treatment.

My oncologist called to report that the consensus of the oncology team was to start me on the Kadcyla and see how I do. Of course, this was not what I wanted to hear. I also learned that you are not supposed to take antioxidants while getting radiation, but I had been taking high-dose vitamin C and lots of other supplements. Despite diligently doing my stretching exercises, I have developed chording on my inner arm. Between having COVID-19, making important decisions about my medical care, and trying to heal myself—it was a lot to juggle!

Post-Op Week Six

As I approached a new chapter in my treatment, it felt like my body just wanted to stop and heal, but I was forcing it into doing things it did not want to do. I needed to decide whether to take Kadcyla and hormone blockers. The basis for switching all patients who have residual cancer from Herceptin to Kadcyla comes from a 2018 study known as the Katherine Study[13].This study concluded that Kadcyla gave patients a 50% decreased risk of reoccurrence as compared with Herceptin alone. If you look at the details, however, that 50% number is misleading. The actual three-year invasive disease-free survival rate in that study was 88.3% with T-DM1(Kadcyla) versus 77% with trastuzumab (Herceptin). That is an 11% difference, not 50%. Prior to 2018, the only drug available for HER2+ patients was Herceptin and many of these patients are still alive 20 years later. Kadcyla increases the risk of neuropathy and low platelet counts, both of which I already had. In fact, 18% of the study participants had to stop the drug due to its side effects.

As Jean-Pierre reminded me, the cure for stage III IBC is surgery, and anything after that is preventative treatment. I had been on Herceptin for six months, and I seemed to be handling it well. Furthermore, I did not fit into the parameters of the study because I was no longer HER2+. For all these reasons, I decided not to switch over to Kadclya, even though the oncologists recommended it. It was a win-win of sorts: They could document in the chart that they recommended the drug so they were off the liability hook and I could continue with the Herceptin.

A month out of surgery and I could finally sleep on my right side. That felt amazing! I have made peace with my disfigurement. Staying in a state of love and grace, I reminded myself that I came into this world flat-chested. The little girl inside of me knows this place and feels safe there, so instead of moving into grief, which I had already worked through prior to surgery, I have been able to let go of what was and accept what is. I started to feel better and stronger day by day. For the first time in a long time, I was on no medication. I always felt better when I wasn't taking any drugs.

In addition to deciding whether to take Kadcyla, I also had to decide whether to go on tamoxifen or another aromatase inhibitor for the foreseeable future. Some of the common side effects from tamoxifen are hot flashes, headaches, fatigue, depression, bone loss, endometrial cancer, and a risk of blood clots. As for aromatase inhibitors, they have the same side effects as tamoxifen plus joint or muscle pain and a greater risk for heart failure and cardiovascular mortality. It goes without saying that all solutions to address any side effects involve taking more medications. And taking those medications was no guarantee that the breast cancer wouldn't return.

There is a Facebook group of women who choose not to take tamoxifen called *Tamoxifen No More*. Most of them went off the drug because of its side effects, and some said their symptoms did not disappear even after they stopped the drug. After reading these posts and seeing the number of patients who suffer from these side effects, one begins to wonder whether the manufacturers claim that only a small percentage of people suffer from these side effects is accurate. Someone should do a study on that! In my case, the tumor was 95% HER2+ and 5% hormone positive. Taking these drugs for five to ten years would only lower my risk of recurrence from 9% to 6%. Is that 3% difference worth the debilitating side effects?

I saw the radiation oncologist and had my mapping procedure. Mapping uses MRI imaging to ensure that all body measurements and calculations are correct prior to starting radiation. The doctor confirmed that the entire torso will be radiated during each session, not just one quadrant, and the rays will penetrate the body from front to back. Due to my skin lupus, he agreed to forgo the seventh week of radiating the scar, a customary practice with IBC patients. When I asked whether I could continue taking high-dose vitamin C while undergoing radiation, he replied that the evidence is mixed and deferred to my judgment. At least he had done his homework!

Post-Op Week Seven

I've been tormented by the possibility that there is that one magic bullet—one thing that prevents cancer's return. Could it be vitamin C infusions, ozone therapy, a keto diet, intermittent fasting, juicing, supplements, or a combination thereof? Why do some people live long lives while other's cancer returns in a year or two? Why do some people eat terribly, refuse to exercise, abuse their bodies, and never get cancer?

Take me, for example: I had little to none of the risk factors that would point to a breast cancer diagnosis, and yet here I sat, facing down another six months of chemo and possibly a decade of hormone drugs. I ate well, was health conscious, not overweight, had no genetic risk factors, exercised regularly, and yet I came down with one of the deadliest versions of one of the deadliest cancers out there!

What is the difference that makes the difference? What is most overwhelming is the sheer volume of information. Among the many Facebook groups of which I am now a member, the books, and the internet or YouTube searches, there is so much information to take in. You feel as though you have to grasp every facet of what is out there, digest it, and incorporate it into your lifestyle - just in order to live!

In a few days, I would begin radiation. I attended a Tong Ren seminar and had an EEM session with Kim, so I felt great. Would these be the last few days of my life that I felt normal? What will happen once I start six weeks of radiation? Will I ever be the same again? I cannot believe I am freely subjecting my poor body to what even my doctor called its "burning and poisoning."

Chapter 9

The Immolation

January 2022

Week One

My radiation treatment was moving forward despite my low blood counts, surgery side effects, and having COVID-19. IBC demands that one does not delay. I was scheduled to receive 30 rounds of radiation over the course of six weeks. Due to my COVID-19 status, I had to sit outside in my car until I was called inside and the staff had to gown up to treat me.

I could drive myself to and from appointments and I was in and out in 15 minutes, but radiation was the most deceptive of all three treatments. It is invisible and silent, but behind its innocuous appearance, it holds the deadliest power.

By Day Two, I was already depressed and feeling sorry for myself. Radiation comes on the heels of two horrific experiences. It breaks down further in the body what has already been damaged or depleted. I was hooked up to a machine in a cold, sterile environment, like a lamb to the slaughter. I could feel my skin shrinking and shriveling as the machine zapped me; it felt like I was being vacuum sealed.

Having to drive there every day was a constant reminder of my diagnosis. After a male technician met me at my car, I went inside and stripped down naked with my one breast exposed and the other missing while three people watched me from another room. Granted, they saw this every day, but for the patient, it is humiliating and dehumanizing. I had not even been able to look at myself in the mirror until earlier that week, and now I was on display for all the world to see.

A part of me was slipping away. I had been battered, broken, and beaten down. How could I hold onto my sense of self when I could no longer remember who I was before this happened? My memory was shot. I felt like a shadow of who I was before all this. I had changed so much; I didn't recognize myself. I jumped a little with fright every time I caught a glimpse of myself in the mirror.

In addition to my daily drives to radiation, I started occupational therapy (OT). The therapist showed me things to do for the scar, but she never touched my body. I thought someone would work on me directly, but apparently, that is not the case. It felt as though I was tasked with having to heal myself.

All day, every day, my time consisted of attempting to manage my symptoms and heal myself. I woke up and did my stretching exercises so my muscles and scar wouldn't stiffen up any further. I put calendula ointment on the scar to keep it moist. I used lymphatic drainage techniques to keep the fluid moving and prevent the chording from getting worse. I did my daily energy exercises to keep my energies from getting scrambled by the radiation.

When I got home from radiation, I put a chamomile tea poultice on the skin to take out the burn. Then I applied aloe vera gel to stop the pain and did the stretching exercises given to me by the OT. It felt like I was my own client, instead of the patient. I was dealing with an emergency that no one knew about but me. And it was only Day Two!

Day Three was even harder than Day Two. It seemed that something profoundly negative energetically happened each time I got radiated. I immediately felt depressed, angry, weak, and vulnerable. I could feel the burn as the radiation was going into my body, and I sensed my energies were getting scrambled, going homolateral and my biofield was collapsing. I asked Kim to test me to see how my systems had been affected. Her testing found these imbalances:

Homolateral - entrenched (See Page 105)

Biofield – obliterated and collapsed (See Page 107)

Chakras – weak and imbalanced (See Page 132)

Scrambled energies (See Page 111)

Shock Points - weak (See below)

Radiant Circuits - offline (See Page 115)

Triple Warmer - reactive (See Page 97)

And this was going to be happening every day!

Releasing Shock From the Body

1. Three points are located vertically on the heel of the foot. The main one is in the center, the other two are equal distance on either side of the main point.
2. Prepare the foot by massaging it on the top and bottom, moving the energy from the heel up through the toes.
3. Press in and apply firm pressure at the middle of the heel for a minute or two.
4. Move to the two other points above and below the center of the heel.
5. You can do both sides at once or one foot at a time.

NOTE: This technique is explained in greater detail on Page 172 .

February 2022

Week Two

I was amazed at how much it felt like I was really on my own trying to navigate my way through this leg of my journey. Maybe it was because I was being radiated at a hospital other than where I received my chemo, but I had yet to see a nurse. I had lots of questions but no one to answer them. Without the IBC Facebook page, I would have really been in the dark. I was concerned because radiation increases one's risk for lymphedema.

At my next OT appointment, I asked the therapist about lymphedema prevention. She said very little research has been done on it and told me about a seminar she attended where a doctor said there is no evidence demonstrating that flying or getting a blood pressure reading on the arm would trigger lymphedema. After he made that statement, three or four professionals in the audience raised their hands and said they had patients whose lymphedema was triggered by those very things—flying and getting blood pressure readings.

The doctor dug in his heels. His position was that because there are no double-blind studies or because the anecdotal evidence contradicts what few studies have been done, the problem does not exist. This is another name for denial. I don't know whether this is due to their medical training or a fear of legal liability, but whatever the cause, this denial prevents patients from getting the information they need. No wonder we have to create Facebook pages to help each other answer the questions that traditional medicine chooses to ignore.

I couldn't take any supplements during radiation, but I was using homeopathic remedies for my side effects. They were definitely helping with the pain and burning. Now that I was finished chemo and surgery, I could take a step back and assess what had transpired until now, at least from an external perspective.

Thanks to the Eden Method, less than a year ago, I had more energy, health, and vigor than the average 64-year-old. I had no pain anywhere in my body: no joint pain, no neck or shoulder pain, nothing. I had no intention of retiring anytime soon. Not even a year later, I felt like I had aged about 15 years. I had substantial joint pain, lower back pain, shoulder pain, and neuropathy. I used to bounce upstairs, never giving a second thought to my footing. Now I had to move slowly and watch my step. Although my hair was finally growing back in and it was soft and curly, it was gray and white—the hair of an old woman. It seemed that whatever side effects I had from chemo, radiation was intensifying or accelerating them.

By the end of Week Two, I had significant neck and right shoulder pain. It was probably from lying on a flat table during radiation treatment and having to raise my arm above my head and not move for 15 minutes every day. Everything felt stiff and tight. The pain woke me up in the middle of the night, so my only recourse was to do energy work. I could easily reach my neurovascular points, so I held stomach, triple warmer and then spleen points.

Holding Stomach Neurovascular Points

1. Place your left hand gently on your forehead.
2. Find the space on the highest point of your cheekbone in line with your right eye.
3. Gently place the pads of your first and second fingers of your right hand on that spot.
4. Hold lightly for several minutes.
5. Switch hands to place your right hand gently on your forehead.
6. Find the space on the highest point of your cheekbone in line with your left eye.
7. Gently place the pads of your first and second fingers of your left hand on that spot.
8. Hold lightly for several minutes.

NOTE: This technique is explained in greater detail on Page 139.

Next, I held my radiant circuit points and finally, my shock points because every treatment was a shock to my body. I didn't know what impact the radiation had on my meridians, but I definitely experienced relief and relaxation on a deeper level after doing these holds.

Week Three

This was the first time I felt pain from the radiation burn. My front chest was red, like skin lupus, but this was not skin lupus. It itched and burned, and there was pus coming out of part of it. The upper back along the scapula was burnt, which surprised me because I didn't realize that much radiation was going there.

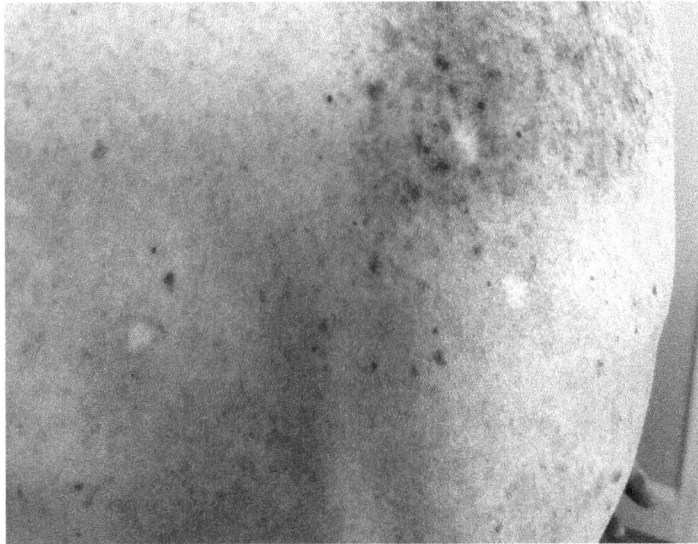

A breast cancer survivor told me to put kale leaves where I was radiated, so out of desperation, after my session, I immediately drove to the supermarket, bought a bunch of kale and put it on my chest. (Do you know how painful that is?!) I had no idea if it worked, but I did it anyway. I added a green tea poultice to my chamomile, aloe, and calendula routine and I was downing homeopathic remedies like they were candy.

At the end of the week, I had a shocking episode while on the table. It felt like the tissue and muscles of my torso were melting into my rib cage. There was pain and numbness along, above, and below the incision that spread to the entire torso. I had a sharp pain shooting up into my armpit. My entire rib cage was inflamed. My lupus might also have been triggered because I had an itchy rash forming at my clavicle. Was this normal for radiation? I decided I better talk to my radiation oncologist. On Thursday, the radiation department called and said not to come in until I had seen the doctor. Four days without a treatment? I felt like I won the lottery. My body could finally get a break!

In the meantime, I had an appointment with a chiropractor who specialized in deep tissue release. He stated that allopathic medical professionals think that when surgery is "successful," that is all that is needed; they don't consider how to restore the tissue, nerves, and muscles that were damaged. He used a technique called *Active Release*[14]. It freed up my pectoral muscle in a way that I could only dream of. By the end of the session, my arm almost felt normal.

Week Four

All the time that I been worried about lymphedema, I should have been worried about radiation fibrosis. Apparently, feeling like I was being vacuum sealed while getting radiated was not normal. I could find scant studies on the impact of lupus or connective tissue disease on radiation side effects, however, there was one confirming that auto-immune illnesses can create acute radiation toxicity and have late effects. It recommended doing a shorter duration of radiation in those instances, but even the study acknowledged that doctors are reluctant to change the way they administer radiation because that's what they have been taught.

Our family engaged in a heated discussion about my treatment. Nurse Nathalie said I should be on Kadcyla and estrogen inhibitors already. She was not happy that I didn't go to radiation on Friday. She said that the side effects I was having were typical and I hadn't been compliant with the normal protocol. She was worried that the cancer would come back because I hadn't been more aggressive.

I, on the other hand, was more concerned about late effects and my long-term quality of life. As much as I didn't want the cancer to return, I could not live the rest of my life taking medications because I was allergic to most of them. Moreover, I had been using so many tools to combat the underlying inflammatory conditions which caused the cancer that I was less concerned about it coming back than about the long-term side effects of treatment. Time will tell which decision was the right one.

I met with the radiation oncologist about my episode on the table. He said my experience was not normal. Our conversation went something like this:

Dr. C: You shouldn't be "feeling" the radiation going in, and you shouldn't be in pain or have new numbness, but I can't take back what happened. You are the boss.

Me: I may be the boss, but you are the expert.

Dr. C: I have to state what the protocol is, but then there is the reality and for someone like you, with auto-immune issues, you might only need three weeks of radiation and not six. Most people feel nothing when they get radiated. It is not normal to feel pain or numbness from the treatment. Even the degree of the burn and the immediacy of the rash is not normal. You are just sensitive to medication and super in touch with your body - which is good. The fact that you responded so strongly is good. I had two patients who did not respond to radiation at all and they both relapsed. I agree that your weight, age and auto-immune issues are all factors that mitigate against doing 30 treatments. I recommend that we hold off on radiating the upper back and scapula and focus on the scar area. Perhaps we could try three sessions this week and reassess on Monday.

Me: Yes, that sounds good.

I was relieved that he listened to me and gave me options. I was worried he would push me and say, you need this regardless of the side effects. He confirmed he too was worried about my skin lupus. It was reassuring to know that to have a skin reaction this fast and this much was unusual.

I went to radiation the next day. My skin started to burn a few hours later, but nothing like the other day. I discovered a whole new problem to be concerned about: radiation recall. It comes after you have finished with radiation and can return months or years later. It is a severe skin reaction to a drug; even a COVID-19 vaccine can trigger it. So can agents of immune therapy, like Herceptin. I hadn't had a Herceptin infusion yet, but I was due for one in a week.

I decided to energy test to ask my body how much more radiation it could tolerate. I tested: 17 days, yes; 18 days, yes; 19 days, started to get weak; 20 days, weaker; 21 days, weak. Between 19 and 20 days maximum. Kim and Jean-Pierre wanted me to stop now. Nathalie was understandably worried about whether it was enough to stop the cancer's return. My research showed a combination of breast cancer and connective tissue disease put me at a greater risk for all post-radiation problems: acute dermatitis, radiation recall, lymphedema, and fibrosis. Radiation was definitely proving to be the hardest part of my treatment.

Week Five

I received my first Herceptin infusion since starting radiation treatment. I felt tired afterwards and went homolateral, but that was not all. For the first time, I truly felt beaten down by this disease. Previously, I was able to bounce back from whatever treatment I was getting with the help of my alternative supports. I might have gone homolateral, but with some effort, I could reverse it. Now, I was under assault: as they say — slashed, burned, and poisoned.

No matter what I tried, I couldn't reverse the homolateral pattern, and my biofield was getting fried every day from the radiation. The burns were getting worse, which was pulling on the incision and, in turn, the pectoral muscle. The radiation burn was just starting and would continue to get worse for the next several weeks. It felt like I was being lanced with a hot poker where my drains were placed.

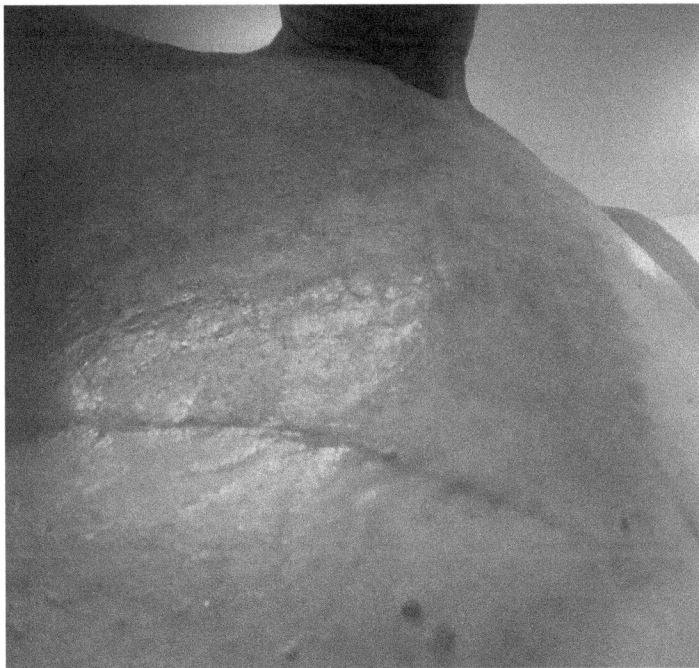

My white and red counts were still low, so that made me tired. My neuropathy was making it hard to walk, so the combination of everything made me feel truly handicapped. Should I stop now or soldier on?

I saw the radiation oncologist and showed him the pus and burn on my torso.

Me: I don't want to radiate that part anymore, just the scar.

Dr. C: I'll have to change the mapping program and I'm not sure I can get it done by the next scheduled treatment. I'll go back to doing the upper back and scapula so that everything will get close to 20 rounds."

Me: Did you have patients who stopped sooner than 30 rounds?

Dr. C: Yes.

Me: Why did they stop?

Dr. C: For the same reason as you.

Me: How are they doing?

Dr. C: Fine. There was a study out of MD Anderson that showed people who had a stronger skin reaction to radiation treatment did better overall.

Me: Ok. Let's do 20 rounds.

Dr. C: Your body will decide.

March 2022

Week Six

By this time, I didn't feel beaten down, I felt beaten up. It was as if someone had kicked me in the ribs. My torso was covered with second degree burns. I could add folliculitis and dermatitis to my list of side effects. I had to cover my chest with a special anti-bacterial gauze to protect the skin and prevent an infection.

In addition to the painful torso, I woke up on Tuesday with a nasty eye infection.

The nurse practitioner thought it was a stye, but Jean-Pierre looked at it and said it was a staph infection secondary to the folliculitis. My immune system was breaking down. It was the cumulative nature of it all that was so debilitating. Yes, that was the word: I felt *debilitated*. It was as if the life force was being sucked out of me.

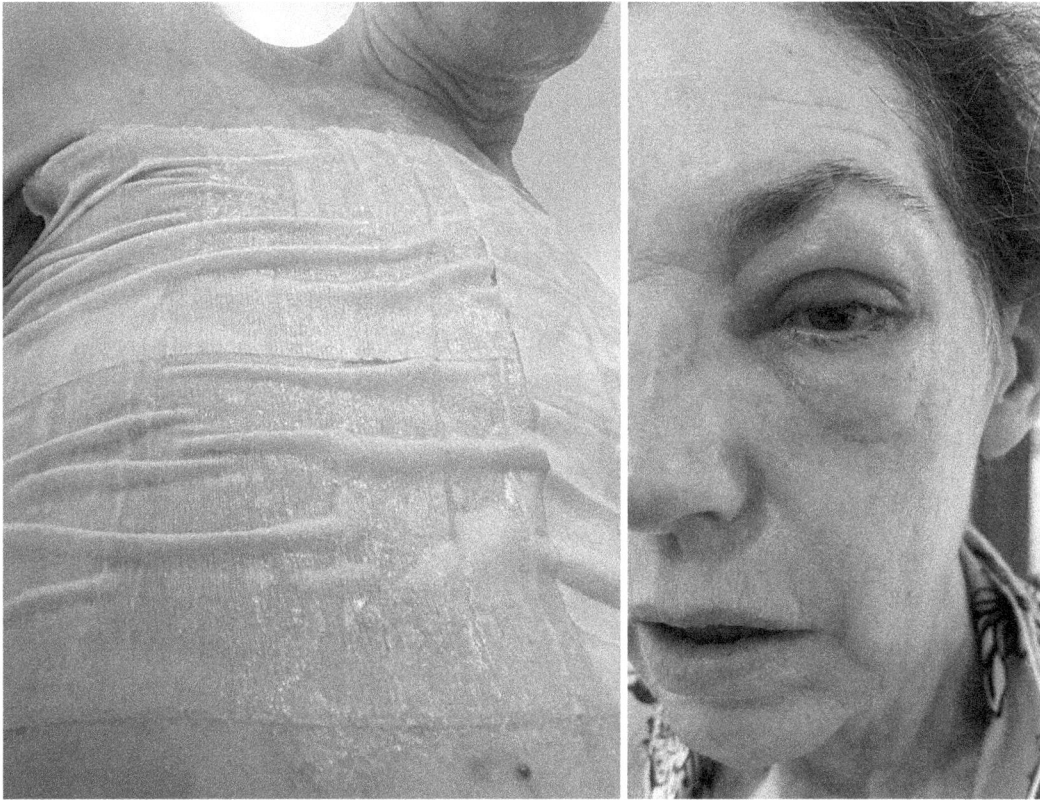

By now, everyone in my family agreed I should stop radiation, but I was determined to reach 20 rounds. I had only one more day to go!

As I was driving up to the cancer clinic the next day, the radiation oncologist called.

Dr. C: You should stop now. Your body is screaming to stop.

Me: Is the pain I am having normal?

Dr. C: No.

Me: Is the redness and inflammation around the area that had just been radiated normal?

Dr. C: No.

Me: How many treatments did I have overall?

Dr. C: Seventeen to the neck and 19 to the lower torso.

Me: I wanted to reach a round number.

Dr. C: That is all your body could take. My goal was to get a reaction from the body and I got it. I wanted to do a good job for you and I feel I've done all that I can and your body is giving a strong signal to stop.

Apparently, a strong skin reaction is indicative of an immune response and therefore a cancer-killing response. Maybe I needed to hear it directly from him so I wouldn't feel guilty for deciding to stop on my own, but my daily trips to the fiery furnace were finally over!

Chapter 10

The Recovery

March 2022

The dreary winter days were ever so slowly becoming longer even if the temperature wasn't budging. Like the frozen earth, I felt numb from all that had transpired. For the first time in nine months, I did not have a Friday appointment for a procedure, test, or treatment. I would continue to have Herceptin infusions for another eight months, but the worst was over. I finally had time to stop and pick up the pieces of what had been a relentless barrage of pain, suffering, and toxicity. Hopefully, time would prove to be the healer and not the revealer of hidden damage.

My last radiation treatment coincided with a Herceptin infusion and it was as if my body had crossed a line from which it might not have been able to return. There was something within me that knew; if I continued to go down that path, there would soon come to be a point in time when it would be too late to come back. Once radiation ended, however, a glimmer of life returned to my body, and it felt like the forces of darkness finally receded. Although my wounds were still fresh and my energy level was low, I had hope that perhaps I could reverse this tide. I could focus on health instead of sickness, and maybe this Humpty Dumpty of a body could be put back together again.

By five days post-radiation, I could feel my skin starting to heal. It was itchy—in a good way. I continued to wear the dressing that protected my skin and helped with the pain. I was grateful for the healing I saw happening so far. I wanted to believe I was out of the woods because, in my mind, I was done. I was not going to take the Kadcyla, Tamoxifen, or aromatase inhibitors, but those were victories in my mind; the battles had yet to be fought. Perhaps I was the only patient who saw cancer treatment to be as much of an enemy as the cancer itself. Maybe it wasn't so much that the treatment was my enemy as much as it was that I had a problem with the one-size-fits-all approach.

I did everything I was told I needed to do to stop the cancer, and now I was unwilling to do anything more that would continue to suppress or damage my immune system. My body needed to heal. It did not need more drugs to dampen and dumb it down. It needed time to rest and find its way back to balance and health. If I entertained the notion of going on an aromatase inhibitor for the next five years, I needed only to read the stories of the women who were in misery due to the side effects of those drugs: constant joint and bone pain, cataracts, permanent tendon damage, weight gain, diabetes, high blood pressure, neuropathy, bone loss, headaches, and hot flashes. My tightrope had now turned into a line drawn in the sand that I would not cross.

I met the oncologist on Friday. She said, "You've been through a lot, haven't you?" She also seemed genuinely surprised that I made it through 19 rounds of radiation. Who knew? The doctors secretly know you might not make it anywhere near the final goal and can adjust for that, yet no one tells you.

Two weeks out, and I believe I was suffering from a bit of PTSD. I broke down in tears when I saw someone I hadn't seen in a year. I felt like I was a mere shadow of who they knew before this war began. I'd start crying at odd times, like going through security at the airport. As often happens in life, we rise to the occasion to fight the foe at our door, but when the danger is over, we collapse. (From an EEM perspective, this often means a Grid has broken, but that's the subject of my next book!)

No one can prepare you for what will happen with a cancer diagnosis: the pokes and prods, the endless appointments, drugs, and tests that wear you down, making you exhausted and numb. Then there is the actual damage to the body that may be permanent. You can only deal with it as it comes at you. You can know about the potential pitfalls and prepare accordingly, but you are walking a treacherous path, and one false move can prove dangerous or even deadly. People say, "Oh, it's only temporary," and that may be true, but it's like saying that being on the frontline of a battlefield is only temporary; the scars remain after the war, and you are not the same person you were when you started. In the old days, they called it "shell shock".

April 2022

A month out from radiation and I had a head cold that moved from my nose to my throat to my chest. I got laryngitis and even felt a bit feverish. How was it that I could be sicker from this cold than COVID-19? Despite the cold, I found I could do more things, but I had to sit down and rest sooner than before. I used to walk by the old folks downtown who sat on the benches for hours and wondered why they did that. Now I know: They are really tired!

My torso was healing nicely. I still put calendula ointment on it daily, but it was no longer constantly nagging me. My pectoral muscle and underarm felt like they were back to where they were before I had radiation so I could do my exercises again. I kept up with my daily temporal tapping mantra:

My body knows how to heal itself from anything.
My body has no trouble healing itself.

I found a wonderful PT who helped me with the chording. She actually touched my body, and it made a world of difference. Getting positive touch while undergoing cancer treatment is critical. I've seen too many clients over the years whose bodies were so traumatized from cancer, they couldn't be touched. Loving touch gives the body a different message from the constant negative poking, injecting, and invasions and allows the sympathetic nervous system to release its grip and relax into a parasympathetic response. I think keeping my energies balanced throughout my treatment with energy work and massage allowed my triple warmer to be open and not shut down so I could receive the benefit of being touched by others.

The large swath of over-the-counter medications I had on my shelf when I started this journey had been replaced with an even larger swath of supplements—all-natural substances.

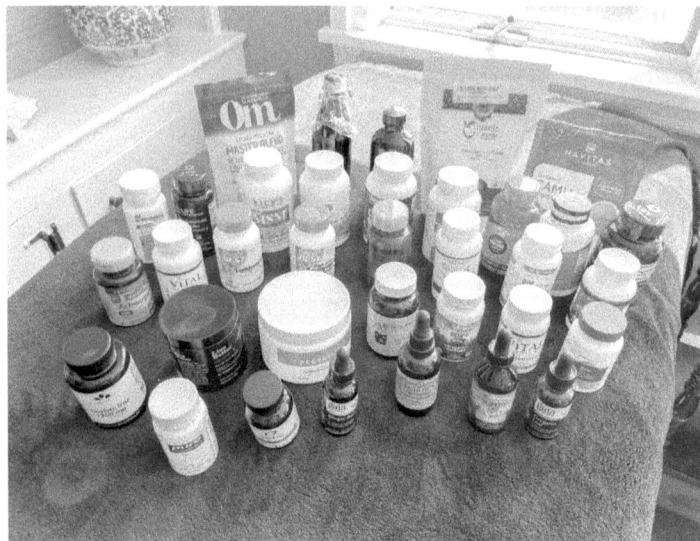

I used them, along with my diet, to detoxify and strengthen my immune system so the cancer would never return. I also joined the Livestrong program at my local YMCA.[15] It is designed for cancer survivors to help them get back in shape and prevent a reoccurrence.

May 2022

I thought I was done, but not so fast. Post-recovery had its own challenges! I seemed to be following the pattern of: two steps forward, one step back. I was struggling with neuropathy and some kind of bone growth in my right foot. My entire right torso was still stiff, painful, or numb. It felt like my chest was sinking or collapsing in spots. Every time I reached for something with my right arm, there was a painful, pulling sensation. My heart had gotten weaker, and exerting myself made it hard to breathe. These were my challenges, but everyone's set of post-treatment recovery is unique. Some late effects are temporary; others are permanent. One's life becomes an adjustment to the new normal.

The psychological fallout was also real. Grief for what has been lost. Depression that one's life and body will never be the same again. Frustration of trying to cope with the new normal. Will my side effects be permanent? Are there other ones waiting down the road? Processing the trauma of what was done to the body and what if the unthinkable happens? What if the cancer returns?

These questions were always lurking in the background and were triggered every time a test, procedure, or medical issue arose. I also had to contend with brain fog and memory issues. Things went in one ear and out the other. I had trouble remembering simple words sometimes and could not remember what happened yesterday. Every Amazon delivery was like Christmas Day: I didn't know what was inside the box until I opened it!

Maybe it was just old age and arthritis kicking in, but I could really see how people get depressed post-treatment with the lingering side effects. One survivor said, "I miss the old me." Well, now I felt like the "old me"; I missed the *real* me.

June 2022

I'd been getting Herceptin infusions every three weeks for nearly a year. Heart damage is the major risk factor for this medication, so an echocardiogram is needed every three months. Until now, I hadn't suffered any apparent side effects from this drug. Lately, however, I'd been having trouble catching my breath after walking upstairs, and my latest echocardiogram showed a significant drop in my left ventricular ejection fraction. This can lead to congestive heart failure, something that runs in my family. The question was: Would this side effect reverse itself once I stopped the infusions or was this a permanent side effect? I decided to stop the infusions until I could consult with a cardiologist.

When I saw the cardiologist, he wasn't as concerned about my left ventricular ejection fraction as he was about my hypertension. I didn't even realize there was a problem. Yes, my readings were in the 170/90s range the last few times I had my blood pressure taken, but it was taken on my leg because it couldn't be taken on my arms. He wanted to put me on medication right away, but I asked if we could just watch it for a few weeks and then decide. Fortunately, it ended up being "white coat syndrome"—that is, it shoots up only when you see the doctor, but I'll never forget what he said at the end of the visit: "People get so caught up in killing their cancer, they forget about the rest of their body and the risks the treatments pose to it."

July 2022

It had been a full year since I was diagnosed. I met the oncologist and asked about my prognosis. Our conversation went something like this:

Dr. V: You have a 60% five-year survival rate.

Me: Why is that?

Dr. V: You only got 19 rounds of radiation.

Me: The radiation oncologist told me I got a good response.

Dr. V: Well, that could have been caused by your skin lupus and was not a therapeutic response. You still had residual cancer in the tumor bed.

Me: Aren't there studies showing that a 95% response is the same as a 100% response in terms of prognosis?

Dr. V: Yes.

Me: Doesn't that give me a better than 60% survival rate?

Dr. V: Yes.

Me: How much better? What percentage?

Dr. V: Somewhere between 60 and 90%, but not above 90%.

I guess I saw that as a challenge and decided I would be part of the 60 to 90% of survivors!

I don't know what the future holds, but the miracle that I hoped for—not having any long-term side effects and not being on any medications for the rest of my life—could possibly be within reach. I am certain that without the support of my family, friends, colleagues, and clients as well as the many modalities I used during my treatment, in particular, EEM, EFT and Tong Ren healing, I would not be in the position I am today: cancer free and free to live my life again!

What follows in Chapters 11 through 15 are energy medicine tips and techniques you and your loved ones can use to help you navigate your cancer treatment. I wish you health and success on your journey!

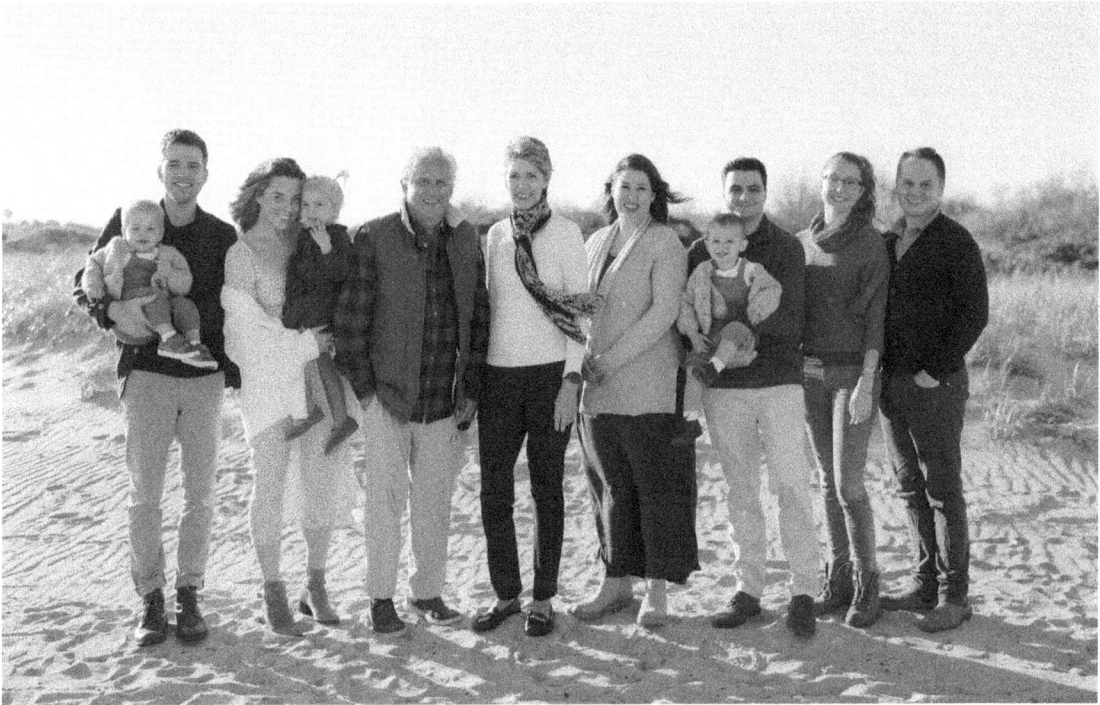

Part II

Mounting a Defense

We make war that we may live in peace.

Aristotle

Chapter 11

Energy Medicine Boot Camp

At an eye exam to assess the need to remove cataracts, it was discovered that one retina had the beginning of macular degeneration. I saw a retina specialist shortly after for an assessment. Following that assessment, I had a session with Dianne, in which she armed me with energy exercises that I could do at home to improve the health of the eye. At my next appointment with the retina specialist, I received a treatment that is known to slow down the advance of macular degeneration. I went back to the retina specialist for a second treatment 6 weeks later. Before the treatment, the doctor was looking at my current retina scan on her screen just below the scan from six weeks prior. She pointed out that the signs of macular degeneration from the previous visit were now gone. She seemed a little puzzled and hesitant. Then she said, "It must be because we caught it early." I received one more treatment that day, and the doctor said that from now on, we would just keep an eye on it, and only do further treatments if the signs of macular degeneration reappeared. A year has passed and I have had regular checkups with the retina specialist. No signs of macular degeneration have recurred.

I am very grateful for the support of Energy Medicine that contributed to the quick disappearance of my macular degeneration.

Jeanne R.

Many people have heard of chakras or meridians, but there are other energy systems I will refer to that are not as commonly known yet they are important to your body's balance. It's helpful to learn how these systems can impact your mind and body so you will understand why a particular exercise is beneficial. In Chapters 12-14, I share exercises that were specific to a particular treatment, but what is described here are the fundamental exercises I needed to do consistently, across the board, regardless of whether I was undergoing chemotherapy, surgery, or radiation.

One of the underlying principles of all energy medicine is that in order to help our body heal, we need to be able to communicate with it. How does one do that? By understanding how the energies move in and around the body and shifting those energies into a healthier pattern.

One simple technique that speaks the body's language is tapping. The body understands and responds to tapping because it mimics the heartbeat. Holding certain acupuncture points on the body is another way of communicating with it. These create space for us to have choices and options as to how we can shift the energies in and around ourselves. For people like me who cannot take medications to counter treatment side effects or for those who prefer to use a more natural method to supplement their allopathic cancer treatment, this next section can help you achieve better overall balance while you undergo your treatment.

Meet Your Commander

Of the nine energy systems in our body, the one that plays a pivotal and perhaps the most preeminent role in our journey is an energy system called *triple warmer*. In TCM, it is known as *triple heater* or *san jiao* meridian as it is viewed as an overarching, unifying force that balances bodily functions like digestion, temperature, heart rate, blood pressure and respiration. The Eden Method, on the other hand, sees triple warmer performing a much deeper and broader role because it is both a meridian and a radiant circuit. Meridians follow fixed pathways in the body and feed an organ associated with it, but radiant circuit energy can move anywhere in the body. Radiant circuit energy is the life force itself and exists in all living organisms. Due to these dual aspects, triple warmer has four functions, including those set forth in TCM; however, it also governs the brain's limbic system, which includes the hippocampus, amygdala, and the fight/flight/freeze aspect of the sympathetic nervous system. Along with spleen meridian, it governs the immune system and the HPA (hypothalamus, pituitary, adrenal) axis, which regulates hormones in the body. Finally, it governs habits in the body. Given these multiple functions, the impact of one facet of this system being out of balance can be enormous.

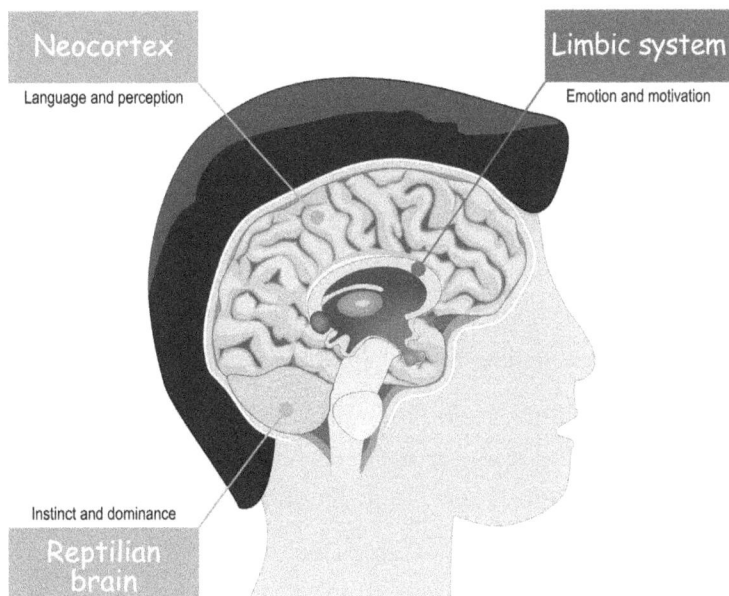

As the commander-in-chief of the body's survival responses, triple warmer will sublimate all other systems of the body—respiration, circulation, reproduction, digestive and immune response—in order to meet the body's perceived real or imagined threat. This stress response, in turn, weakens not just the immune system, but potentially other bodily functions as well. At least 80 to 90% of all illnesses can be tied to stress response in the body. At the heart of most diseases, whether it be cancer, allergies, or autoimmune disorders, there is an overabundance of triple warmer energy in the body. Calming this overreaction is key to bringing the body and its functions back into balance.

If stress is unaddressed over a prolonged period of time, the body can get "stuck" in this over-reaction status. A perfect example of this is PTSD. The body has suffered some kind of trauma and it continues to react as though the trauma is ongoing. A cancer diagnosis and its treatment are traumas to the body. In EEM, this is called *triple warmer reactivity.* Psychologists are beginning to realize that talk therapy alone is not effective to resolve most anxiety or PTSD conditions because they now understand that trauma is trapped in the nervous system, cells, and tissues of the body. Talk therapy, which uses the prefrontal cortex to resolve issues, cannot reach traumas that are being driven by the emotional brain (limbic system). This is the part of the brain that is controlling the sympathetic nervous system, that is, the body's fight/flight or freeze response.

If we take an energy medicine approach to these stressors, it is important that we develop a relationship with our triple warmer energy because it is in the driver's seat. The bad news is, because it governs the limbic brain, triple warmer is not very bright. You can't use reason or logic to motivate or move it. I like to think of it as a small child or a dog. It's often on autopilot based upon our past experiences, which laid down the neural pathways that created the stress loop in the first place. The good news is that it's not very bright. Like a small child or a puppy, it can be trained to change its behavior, but you must first learn how to speak its language. And like a small child or a puppy, successful learning depends on repetition.

Once you learn its language, you can give your triple warmer direction, and it will follow your command. In fact, like a dog, its job is to protect us, and it will calm down only when it feels our body is safe. So, if you stop and think about any medical test, procedure, or surgery you might be undergoing from your triple warmer's perspective, it will be perceived as an assault or direct attack on your body. The limbic system cannot comprehend that a particular procedure is in your best interest; it will react on a subliminal level as if your life is under threat. Have enough of these tests, procedures, or surgeries and your body will have trouble bouncing back. As one survivor stated, "They cured my cancer, and I am 20 years post-treatment, but my body never recovered from the treatment."

How do we keep our mind and body resilient, so it can bounce back from treatment? We must establish a relationship with our triple warmer system and communicate with it so it doesn't get stuck in a fight/flight/freeze reaction. The following exercises helped me whenever I found myself feeling anxious or reactive.

Triple Warmer Reactivity Holds

Triple Warmer Neurovascular Hold

When: Prior to and after a procedure, test, or treatment. Anytime you feel stressed out or overwhelmed.

Why: When the body goes into stress response, blood, oxygen, and energy move out of the brain and into the extremities in order for the body to fight (arms) or flee (legs). There are acupuncture points on the head called *neurovascular points*. These points calm an emotional stress response in the body. They give the brain a different signal and allow the blood, oxygen, and energy to remain in the head so the sympathetic nervous system doesn't need to kick in and flood the body with stress chemicals. They balance the energies between the limbic and prefrontal parts of the brain so the executive functions of the brain can respond to the stressor without getting shut down by triple warmer.

How: Be sure that when you do this exercise your hands are *lightly* touching your head. You don't want to compress your hands on the head, or it will block the flow of blood, oxygen, and energy.

1. Place one palm of your hand on your forehead and the other on the back of your head directly behind your eyes.
2. Breathe in through your nose and out through your mouth.
3. Shift your breathing so your exhale is slightly longer than your inhale. For example, if your normal rhythm is a five-count breath, inhale to the count of five and exhale to the count of six. This helps to shift the nervous system into a parasympathetic response (rest and digest). Closing your eyes will also help.
4. You can lie down with your arms propped up on pillows if your arms get tired.
5. Hold this pose for at least three minutes or until you find your body releasing its stress response.

How will you know when that is? Some people sigh, others yawn. Or, surprisingly, you might find that it becomes harder to think of what it was that was stressing you out in the first place!

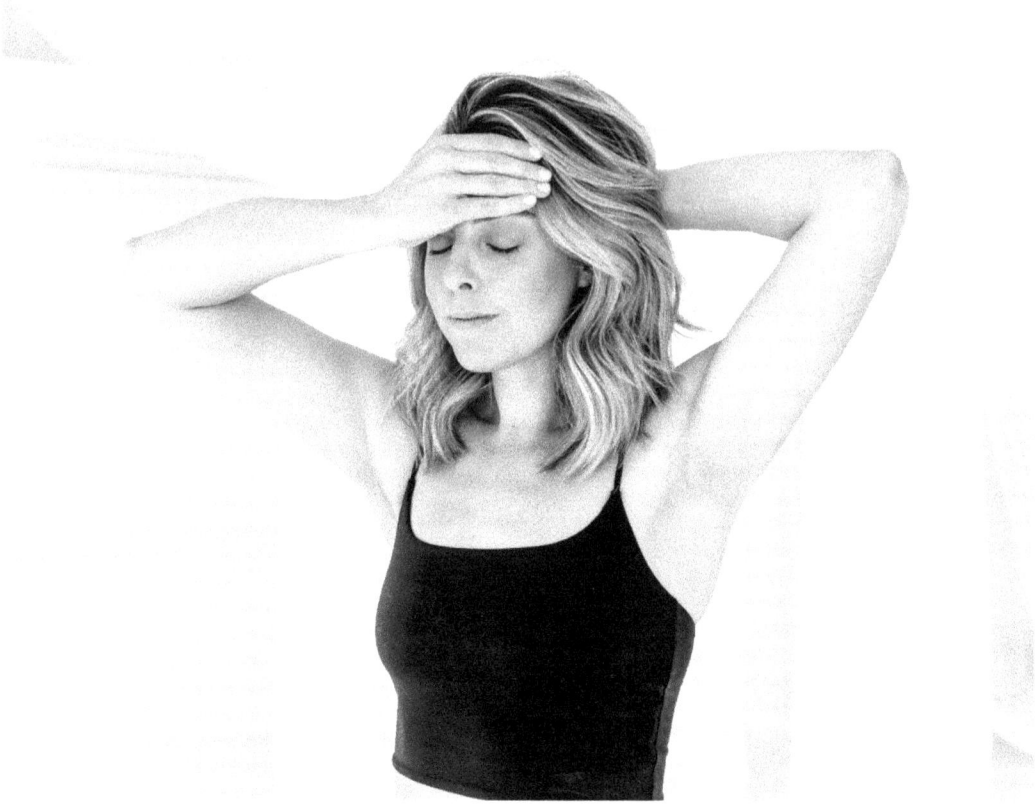

Triple Warmer Mudra Hold

When: Prior to and after a procedure, test, or treatment. Anytime you feel stressed out or overwhelmed. This exercise was designed to address triple warmer reactivity (PTSD) in particular.

Why: In addition to keeping the blood, oxygen, and energy from flowing to the extremities, holding the fingers in this specific configuration gives a direct message to triple warmer. Each finger is the beginning or endpoint of a meridian. The pointer finger is the beginning of the large intestine meridian, which involves holding on and letting go in the body, both literally and figuratively. When you place your pointer finger on your temple, you are having a conversation with your triple warmer because the temple region is the endpoint of the triple warmer meridian. Holding this pose tells triple warmer to *let go* of its overenergized response. The other three fingers placed across the forehead comprise all three fire elemental meridians—the middle finger is pericardium; the ring finger is triple warmer, and the little finger is the small intestine and heart. Holding these three fingers lightly across the forehead calms the entire fire element which, if out of balance, creates anxiety and panic.

In TCM, bladder meridian governs the nervous system so placing the little finger at the inner eyebrow helps calm the nervous system because bladder meridian runs through that point. Placing the middle finger across the center of the forehead calms the main neurovasculars which govern emotional stress. Placing the middle fingers at the hairline touches the liver neurovascular points which help balance stress hormones. So, this hold is a more sophisticated, deeper conversation with your triple warmer.

How:

1.   Make an OK sign with your thumb and pointer finger.

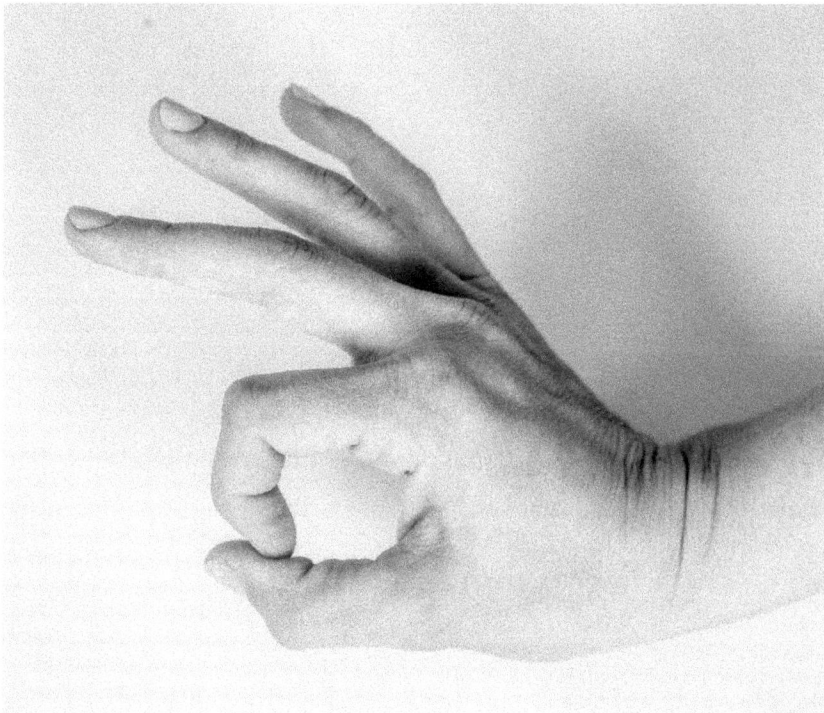

2.   Turn your hand and place the tip and middle portion of your pointer finger directly on your temple. Your thumb will function to support the pointer finger.

3. Place the three remaining fingers across your forehead. The little finger should rest on the inner edges of the eyebrows, the ring finger should rest across the center of the forehead and the middle finger should rest at the hairline. Remember to hold these fingers with very little pressure on the forehead.

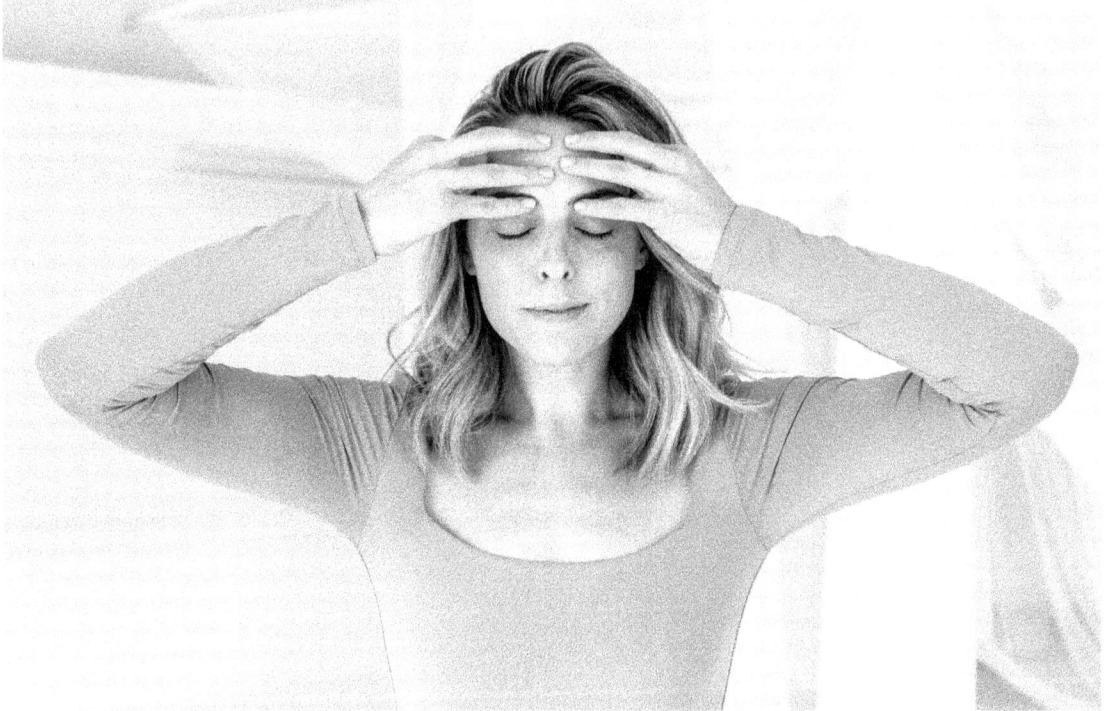

4. Inhale to the count of five and exhale to the count of six: in through your nose and out through your mouth. If you can, place your tongue at the base of your mouth. Doing so gives the sympathetic nervous system the message that it is safe.
5. You can lie down with your arms propped up on pillows if your arms get tired.
6. Hold for at least three minutes or until you feel your body calming down.

People ask, "How long do I need to do these exercises before I see a change?" In many cases, it will be immediate. For others, it might take some time to "reprogram" the nervous system. Using our puppy analogy, how has your puppy been treated? Does it have a history of abuse, neglect, or illness? What breed is it? What is its temperament? To complicate things further, because triple warmer governs habits in the body, entrenched patterns can take some time to reverse and repattern. This puppy can be retrained, however, and taught a different way to live.

Triple Warmer Tracing

Just as there may be 50 ways to leave your lover, there are probably 50 ways to calm triple warmer, too. Why? Because, as keeper of the habits, triple warmer can sometimes become resistant to change, so having lots of tricks up one's sleeve can help keep it resilient and flexible.

When: Anytime you feel stressed. This one is simple and can be done while sitting in a doctor's office or watching TV. I used this exercise continuously when I first discovered EEM. At the time, I was allergic to allergy medications and was suffering from seasonal allergies. This was all I could do, and I did it whenever possible. Within a few weeks, my allergy symptoms were gone.

Why: Even though triple warmer is both a meridian and a radiant circuit, we can impact it by working with the meridian alone. Each meridian flows in a specific direction. When triple warmer has too much energy, we want to take energy out of the meridian. This is done by tracing the meridian in the opposite direction in which it normally flows. This, in turn, sedates the meridian and calms the stress response.

How: The meridian starts at the tip of the ring finger, moves up the top of the forearm to the elbow, up the back of the arm, across the shoulder, behind the ear, and ends at the temple.

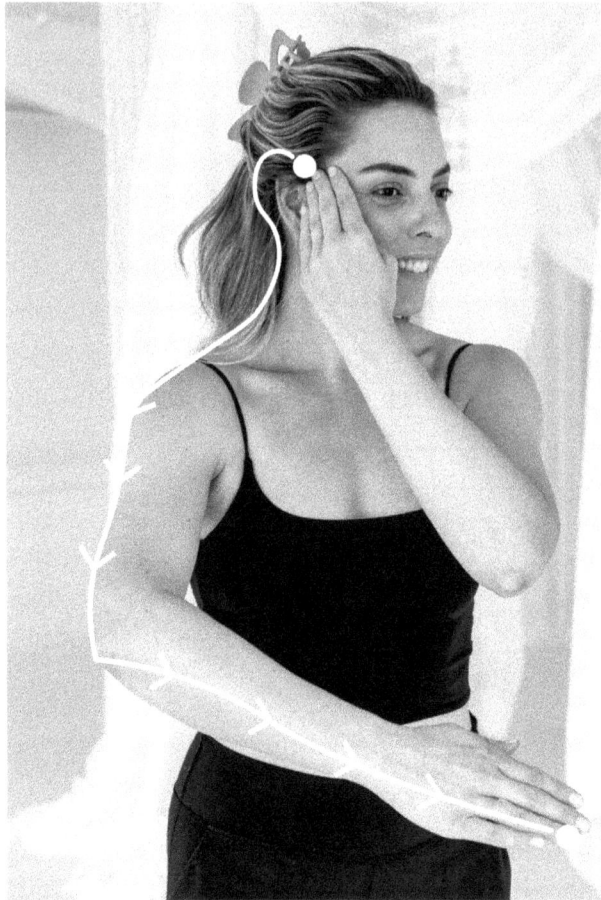

1. Using your left hand, start at your right temple and trace the meridian backwards, behind the ear, across the shoulder, down the back of the arm to the elbow, across the forearm and off the ring finger.
2. You can use your full hand or your little finger (heart meridian). Doing this slowly will further help calm stress response in the body. Thinking about our puppy analogy again: Dogs love being petted because we are essentially tracing their triple warmer meridian backwards!
3. Do this as many times as you feel is needed. Then do the left side of the body.

Combat Retraining

Crossover patterns can be found throughout the body, starting at the microscopic level in our DNA structure to the macro level at the optic chiasm, where the optic nerve connects to the brain. From an energetic perspective, the health of the body is reflected in the degree to which there are strong crossover patterns in and around the body. Another fundamental crossover pattern of our body exists in the connection between the brain's right and left hemispheres.

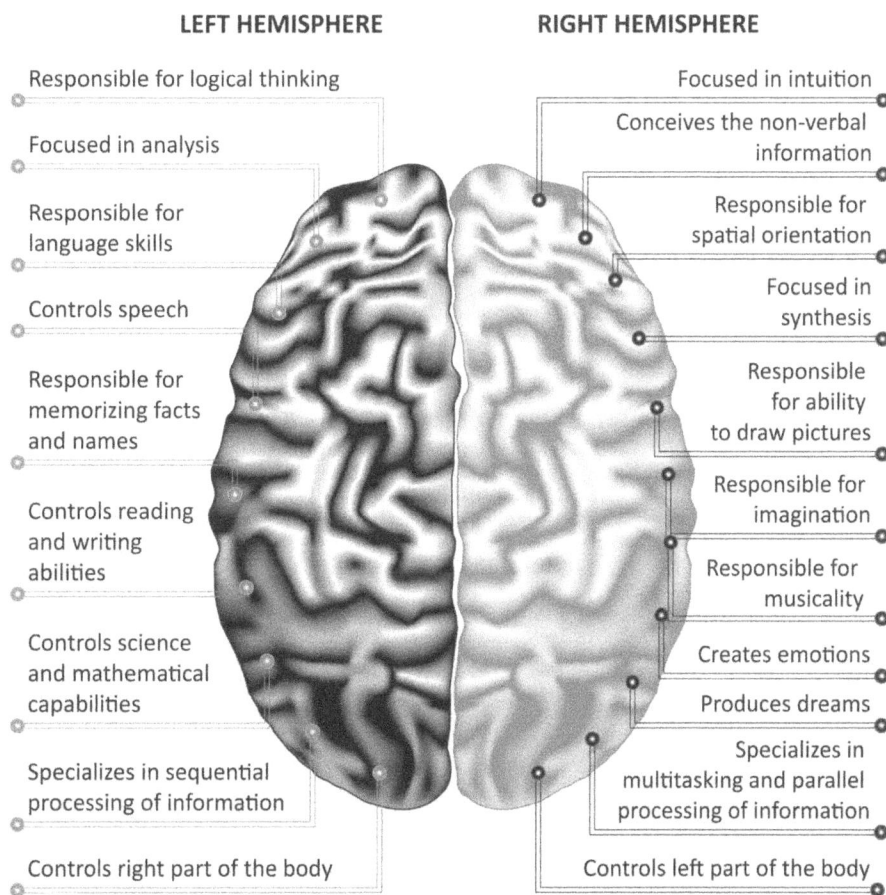

LEFT HEMISPHERE   **RIGHT HEMISPHERE**

Responsible for logical thinking   Focused in intuition

Focused in analysis   Conceives the non-verbal information

Responsible for language skills   Responsible for spatial orientation

Controls speech   Focused in synthesis

Responsible for memorizing facts and names   Responsible for ability to draw pictures

Controls reading and writing abilities   Responsible for imagination

                        Responsible for musicality

Controls science and mathematical capabilities   Creates emotions

                        Produces dreams

Specializes in sequential processing of information   Specializes in multitasking and parallel processing of information

Controls right part of the body   Controls left part of the body

This communication is created via the corpus collosum, where neural pathways start to develop when a baby begins to crawl. It is an important milestone in brain and body development. Prior to this stage of development, the energies run homolaterally and do not cross over.

Because this homolateral condition is innate and the crossover brain pattern is created only via effort, when the body is stressed, the brain will revert to its default pattern, the homolateral condition. When stressed, whether it is from an illness, medical procedure, or something else, the body will attempt to slow down and shut down that communication so it can heal. Using our puppy analogy again, when an animal gets sick, it tends to crawl into a corner and rest. This is part of nature's design, but it should only be a temporary state while one is healing.

What can happen over time, however, is that the homolateral pattern can become entrenched and the mind and body then have difficulty moving back to a healthy state. How do you know if you are homolateral? You can energy test yourself, but symptomatically, it manifests as feeling lethargic, depressed, and unable to heal or move forward in life. The classic couch potato is another symptom: you know in your mind what you need to do, but you just can't muster the energy to do it. This is a *de facto* homolateral pattern. If you are feeling sorry for yourself, depressed, or feeling like a victim, this is another clear sign that your energies have gone homolateral. Similarly, if you exercise and feel more tired afterwards, your energies are probably running homolaterally.

Because triple warmer governs habits in the body, this homolateral pattern can become persistent over time. Counteracting this pattern is one of the keys to staying healthy and resilient in the face of chronic illness or stress. The following exercises can help to shift one's energies out of a homolateral state back into a contralateral pattern. This, in turn, helps the body come back into balance, reconnects the brain's right and left hemispheres, and sets up the conditions for the body to begin to heal from whatever trauma it has encountered.

Contralateral Corrections

Homolateral Repatterning

When: Before and after you have had a test, procedure, or treatment. Remember, your triple warmer perceives anything done to the body as a threat at the subliminal level. Chances are that a stress response will trigger a homolateral condition. I found during my treatments that I went into a homolateral condition sometimes multiple times a day, depending upon what my body was experiencing.

Why: Because homolateral energy is the default pattern in the body, it can be difficult for you to move out of it. Many people live their lives stuck in a homolateral energetic pattern and believe it is their personality. It is not: it is their energy pattern. Moving out of this pattern will help the body heal from whatever it has encountered in life. It can take some time for this pattern to be retrained; however, eventually the body will get the message and hang onto the crossover pattern. You will just feel more energy, more clarity of mind, and less fatigue.

How: This is a good example of how to retrain our puppy. It may have learned one pattern, but we want to teach it something else. Rather than taking a heavy-handed approach, we will gently coax it to adopt a new pattern. First we want to replicate the homolateral pattern and then shift it slowly into a crossover pattern. This exercise can be done standing up, sitting down, or even lying down.

1. Start by tapping your right hand to your right knee and your left hand to your left knee. Do this ten times.
2. Next, tap your right hand to your left knee and your left hand to your right knee. Do this ten times.
3. Repeat the first and second steps two more times. Be sure to cross the midline of your body when you do the crossover tapping so your body gets the clear message that its energies need to start crossing over.
4. End with ten more crossover taps on each side of the body. This final set of crossover taps is what reinforces the message you want to give the body to stay contralateral.

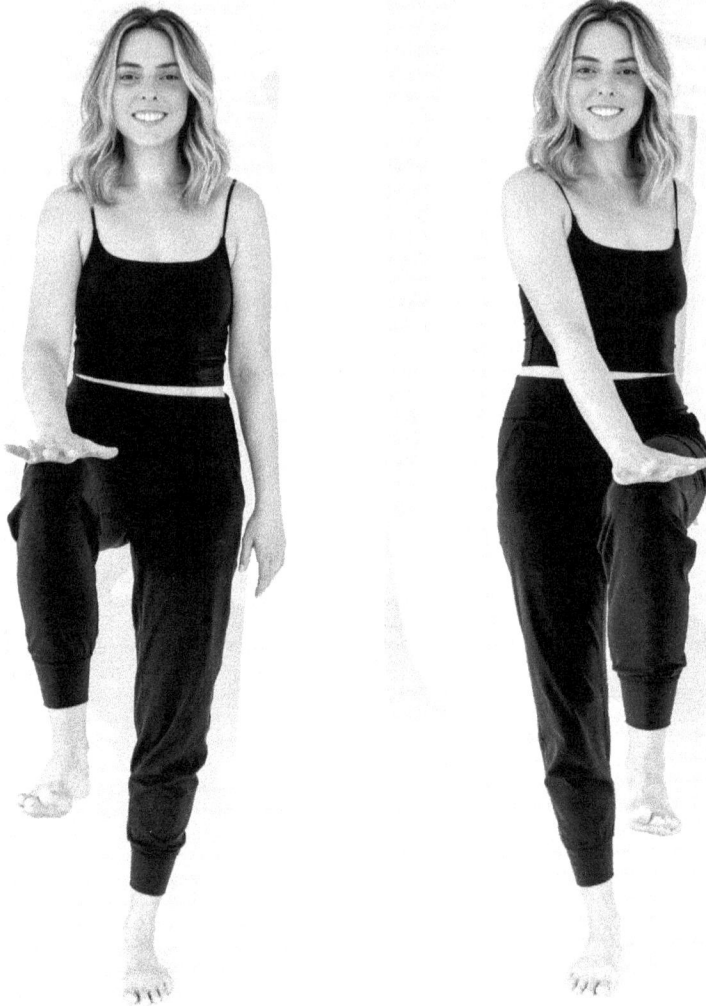

5. If you cannot muster the energy even to do this exercise, you can do the following: Using your pointer finger (large intestine meridian again) trace figure eights around your eyes slowly as if you are drawing glasses on your face. Do this for at least one minute.

6. Do these exercises several times a day until your body can hold the pattern.

The Celtic Weave

When: Whenever your space has been invaded, whether it be a test, procedure, or treatment. Whenever you are feeling unsafe or vulnerable.

Why: This exercise builds and reinforces an energy system that Donna Eden calls the *Celtic Weave*, a webbing that holds all the energies of the body together. It sits inside of the biofield, another one of the nine energy systems of the body. Like the earth's atmosphere that shields and protects it from toxicity, the biofield protects the body from outside toxins and illnesses. Anytime you have a test or procedure that directly impacts the body (MRI, CT scan, etc.), it can create a disturbance in the biofield, including holes or tears in the field. Doing this exercise will help to restore your biofield to a healthier state and protect your body from environmental vulnerability. Aim to do this twice a day and/or whenever something affects your body directly.

How: You want to be standing up for this one, but if you can't stand, it's OK to sit:

1. Rub your hands together and then shake them off.
2. Inhale and place your hands next to your ears.
3. Exhale and cross your arms in front of your chest.

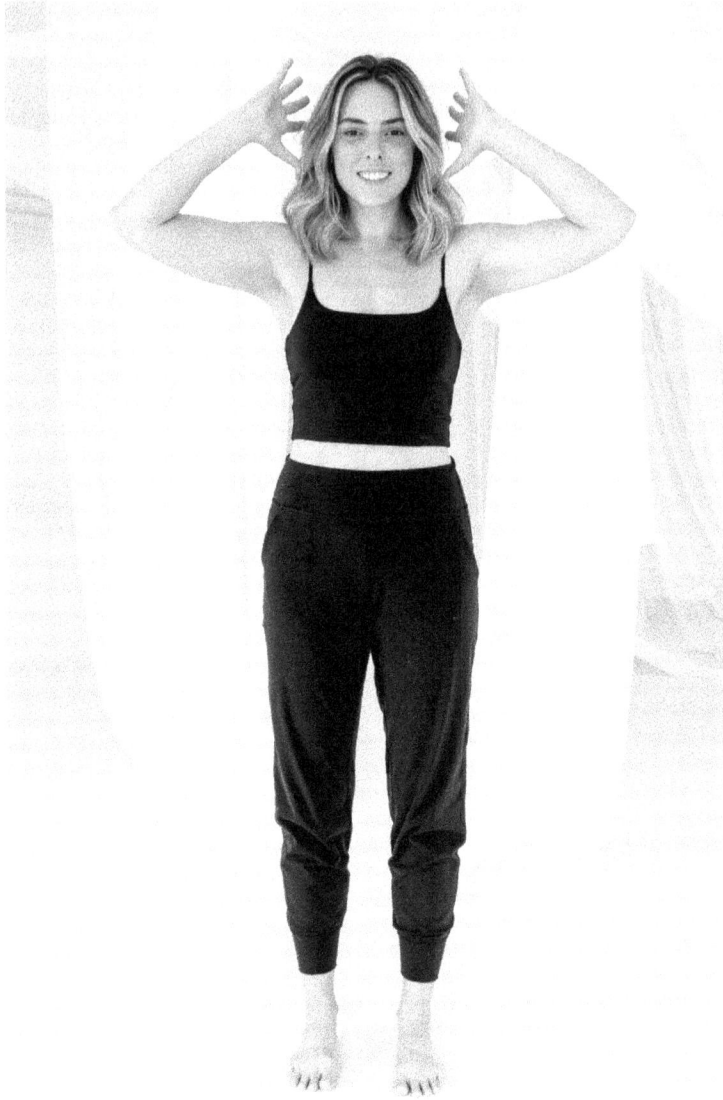

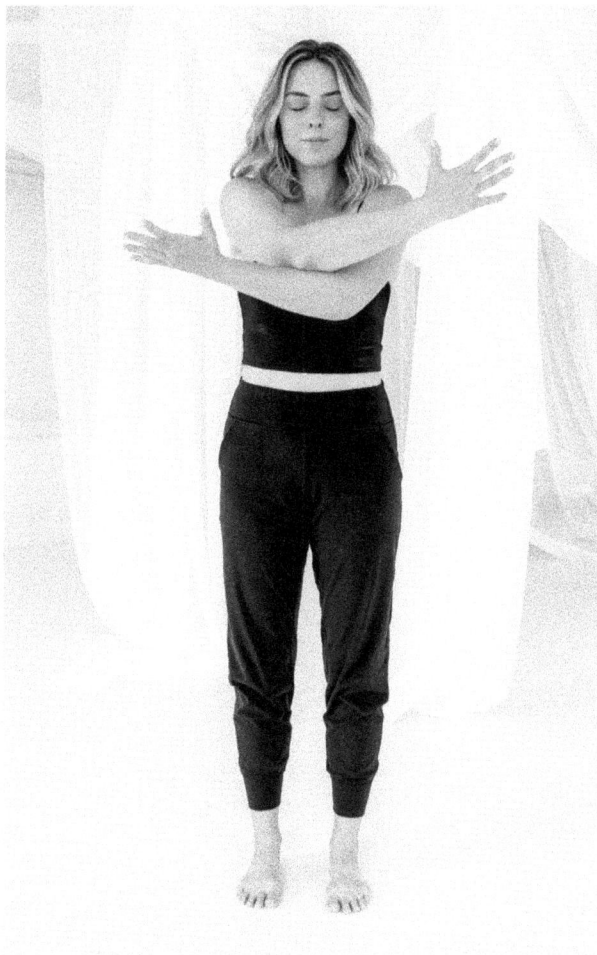

4. Inhale and extend your arms away from your body out to the sides.

5. Exhale and cross your arms in front of your waist.

6. Inhale and extend your arms away from your body out to the sides.

7. Exhale and cross your arms in front of your knees.

8. Inhale and expand your reach away from your body to the sides.

9. Exhale as you approach your feet and reach your hands behind them. Scoop and bring the energy up the front of your body and imagine you are feeding the energy all around your biofield.

10. Expand your arms above your head and out to the sides.

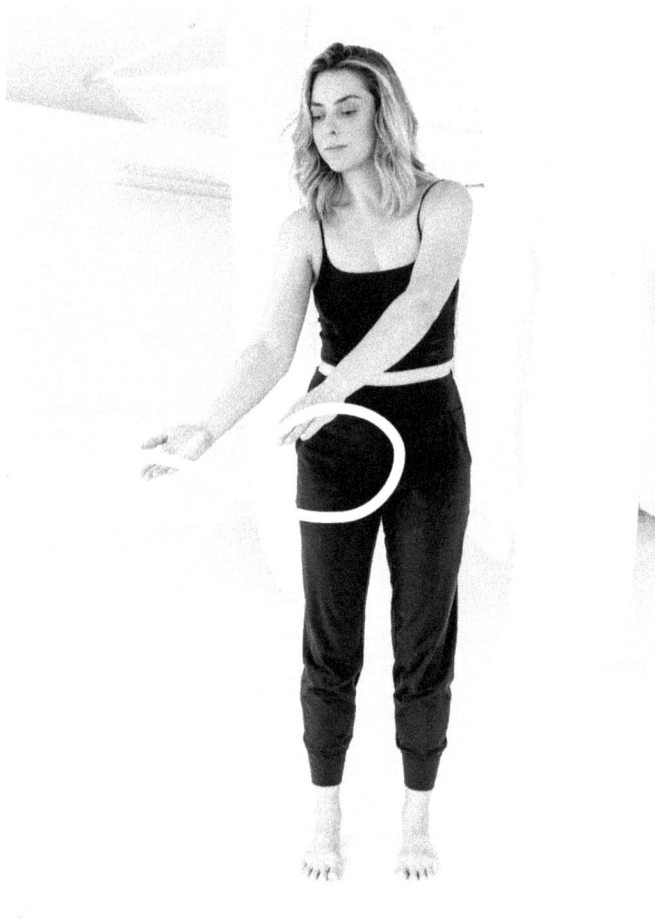

11. End by making large figure-eight crossovers all around your body: in front, in back, on the sides, and so forth. There is no wrong way to do this—as long as you are making crossover patterns with your hands and arms, you're having an impact.

12. Do the exercise a second time.

Cook's Crossovers

When: Whenever you feel overwhelmed, unable to think clearly or if your memory is faltering. In EEM vernacular, this is known as "scrambled energy". In the same way that the right and left hemispheres become energetically vulnerable under stress, the front and back brain also become imbalanced with the limbic system kicking into high gear and the prefrontal cortex shutting down. This can affect one's ability to think clearly. The gut punch one feels when learning of a cancer diagnosis is an extreme example of scrambled energy.

Why: Just as we started retraining triple warmer when we did the homolateral correction, this exercise reinforces crossover patterns throughout the body. Holding the ball of the foot strengthens the kidney meridian, which is the meridian from which chi starts to flow throughout the body. It is also grounding. Holding the points on the forehead reinforces the pineal gland, the sixth chakra, and the corpus collosum—the nexus between the right and left brain hemispheres. Dragging your fingers out to your temples calms triple warmer as does tracing it backwards. Ending at the heart gives your triple warmer the message to move its focus away from the brain and into the heart center.

How: This exercise should be done sitting down.

1. Cross your right leg over your left knee so your right foot is supported by the left knee.
2. Place your right hand over the ball of your left foot.
3. Place your left hand around the top of your right ankle. Your arms will be crossed over each other.
4. Sit up as straight as you can and take five inhales through your nose and exhale through your mouth.

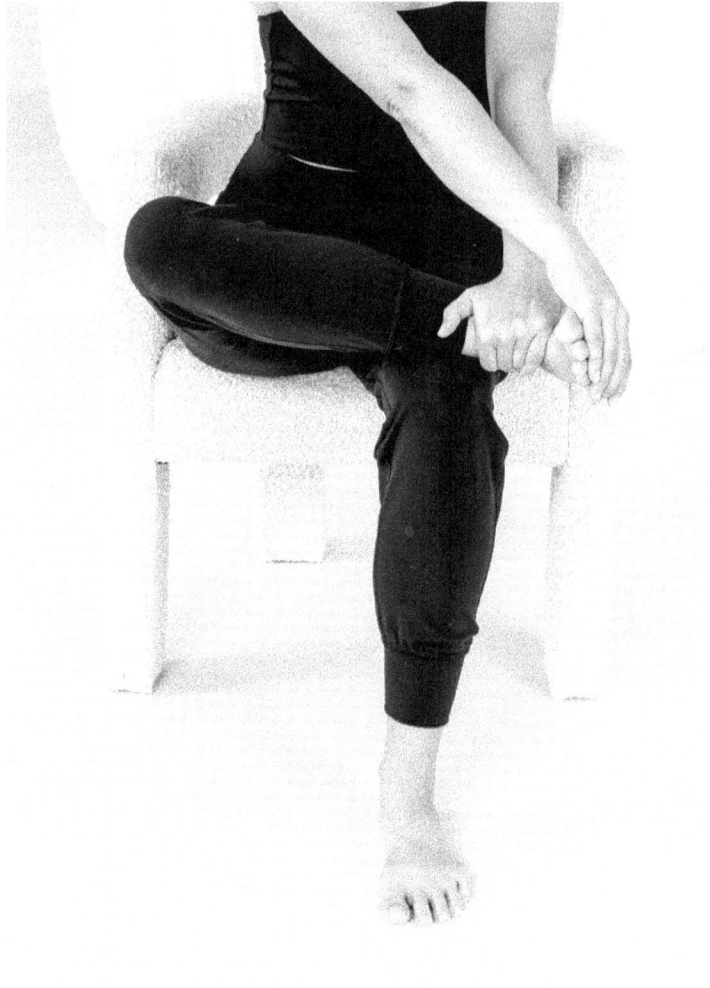

5. Now switch sides and cross your left leg over your right knee.

6. Place your left hand over the ball of your right foot.

7. Place your right hand over your left ankle.

8. Take five breaths.

9. Now steeple your fingers and place your thumbs in the middle of your forehead (at the third-eye chakra).

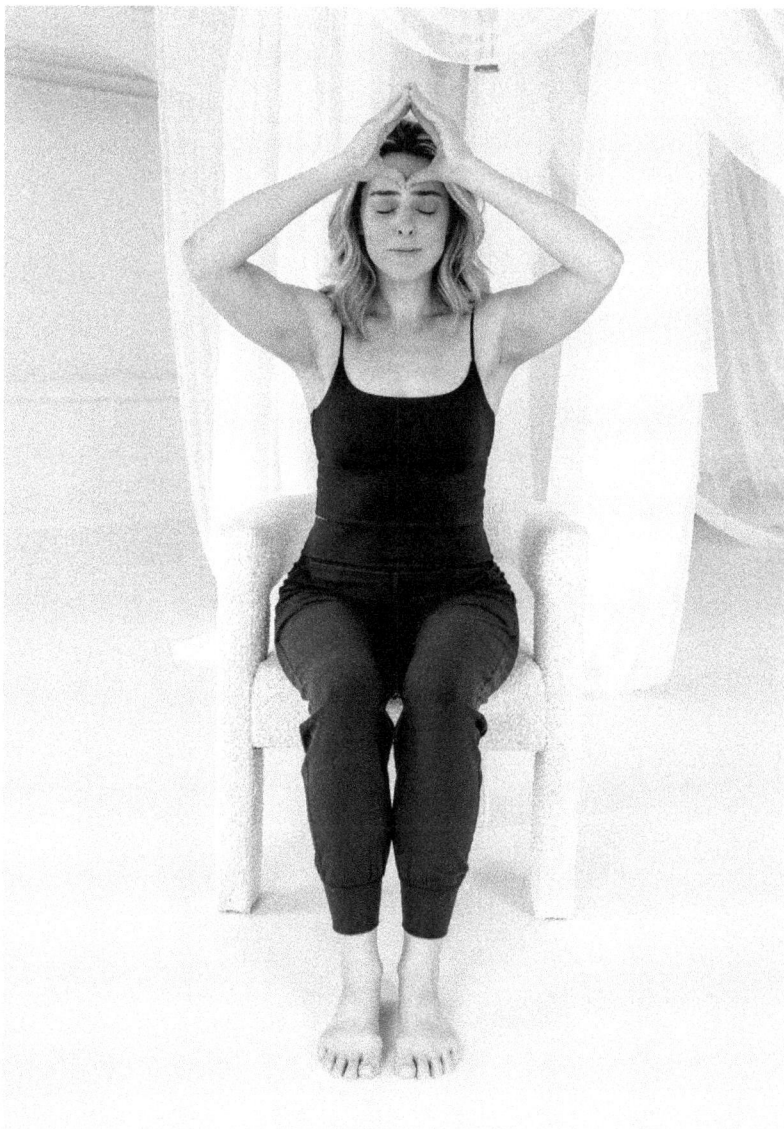

10. Take another five breaths.

11. Place your fingertips where your thumbs were and drag your fingers out to your temples on the inhale.

12. Exhale and draw your fingers up over the backs of your ears to trace the triple warmer meridian backwards.

13. End by placing your hands over your heart chakra.

Bringing in the Big Guns

Radiant circuit energies are another one of our nine energy systems. Donna Eden calls them *radiant circuits* because they bring radiance and healing to the body. In TCM, they are known as either "strange flows" because they don't follow the regular patterns of meridians or "extraordinary vessels" because they can go anywhere in the body where healing is needed once activated.

Anytime you focus on the beauty of a sunset, listen to peaceful music, or meditate, you are touching into radiant circuit energy as this energy system is strongly impacted by positive emotions like joy, love, and gratitude. The Eden Method views triple warmer as a meridian and a radiant circuit because it can go anywhere in the body when it perceives a threat to your survival (with the exception of the heart because the pericardium protects the heart).

Consequently, working with radiant circuit energies can have a double benefit: It can calm the body's stress response, and it can help the body heal. Just as the body can go homolateral due to an illness or too much stress, the radiant circuit energies can go dormant and stop providing their abundant healing services. By holding certain points along their flows, we can preserve or reactivate their circuitry.

Radiant Circuit Holds

Yin and Yang Bridges

When: I would do these techniques when I was too sick to get out of bed. I found that by holding these points, I was able to heal faster from whatever it was I was encountering, whether it be nausea from chemo, pain from surgery, or fatigue from radiation. I often held them if I couldn't sleep and found it would help me fall back to sleep.

Why: As mentioned above, the radiant circuit energies can go dormant in the body. Cancer treatment is a repeated trauma to the body and over time can cause this primary energy system to shut down. This can explain why some people may be declared "cancer free" but never really recover from their treatment, either mentally or physically. Those lingering, residual side effects take prominence in their lives because their radiant circuit energies have stagnated.

How: These holds can be done sitting up or lying down. To tune into the full benefits, close your eyes while doing them. This is also a wonderful treatment for a loved one to perform. You want to be comfortable because you will be holding these points for a while. Don't think about how long to hold them; the longer you hold them, the more they will become activated. If you tune into your body, after several minutes you may start to feel peaceful as these flows start to stir deep inside.

1. Place your fingers or full hand over the circle point. You may hold any of the circled points.
2. Place your other hand anywhere along the circuit line you can easily reach. If you can place your arm along the line, that's even better, but don't strain.
3. Try to have your hands crossing to the opposite side of the body.
4. Hold these points for at least three to five minutes or as long as you wish. The longer you hold them, the deeper it goes.
5. After holding the circuit point and circuit line, switch hands and hold on the opposite side of the body.

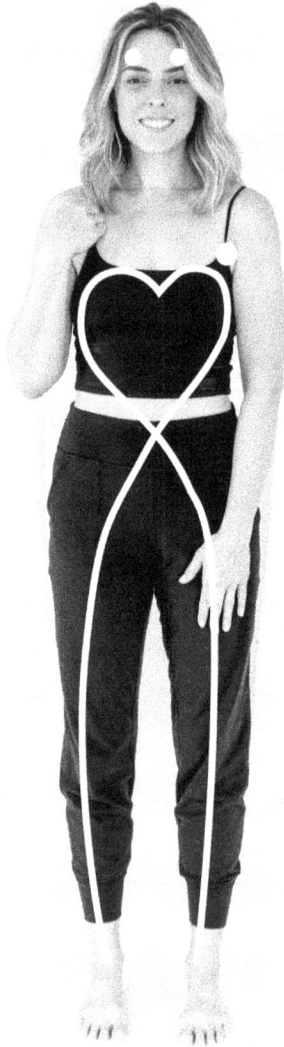

Yin Bridge Hold

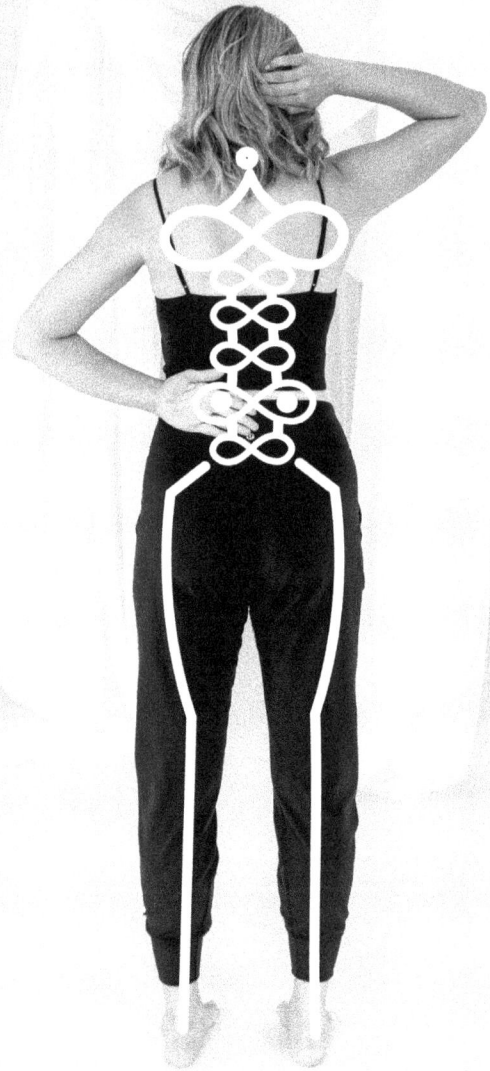

Yang Bridge Hold

Yin and Yang Regulator Poses

When: Same as yin and yang bridge holds above.

Why: Same as yin and yang bridge holds above. The regulator flows govern all systems in the body: circulation, hormones, digestion, and so forth. Holding these points can help address any global issue one might be experiencing and bring healing energy to that system.

How: Same as the yin and yang bridge holds above.

Yin Regulator:

1. Place your right hand on the right side of your forehead in line with your right eye and your left hand somewhere along the inside of your left leg.

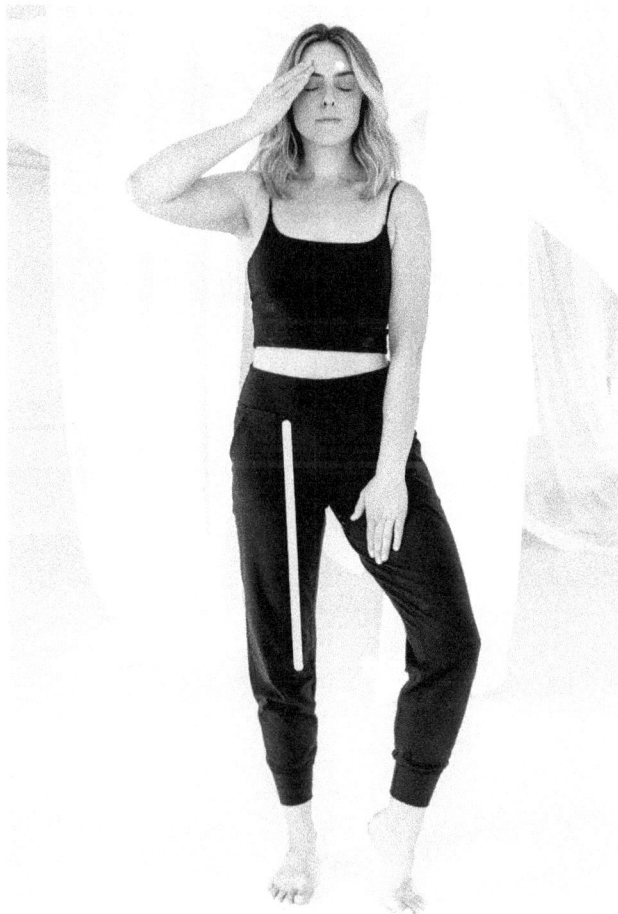

2. Hold these places for at least three to five minutes.

3. Switch sides and place your left hand on the left side of your forehead in line with your left eye and your right hand along the inside of your right leg.

4. Hold these places for at least three to five minutes.

Yang Regulator:

1. It's easiest to turn on your left side and place your right hand under your left arm where the arm meets the torso.

2.   Place your left arm along the lateral side of your left leg (where the outside seam of your pants would run).

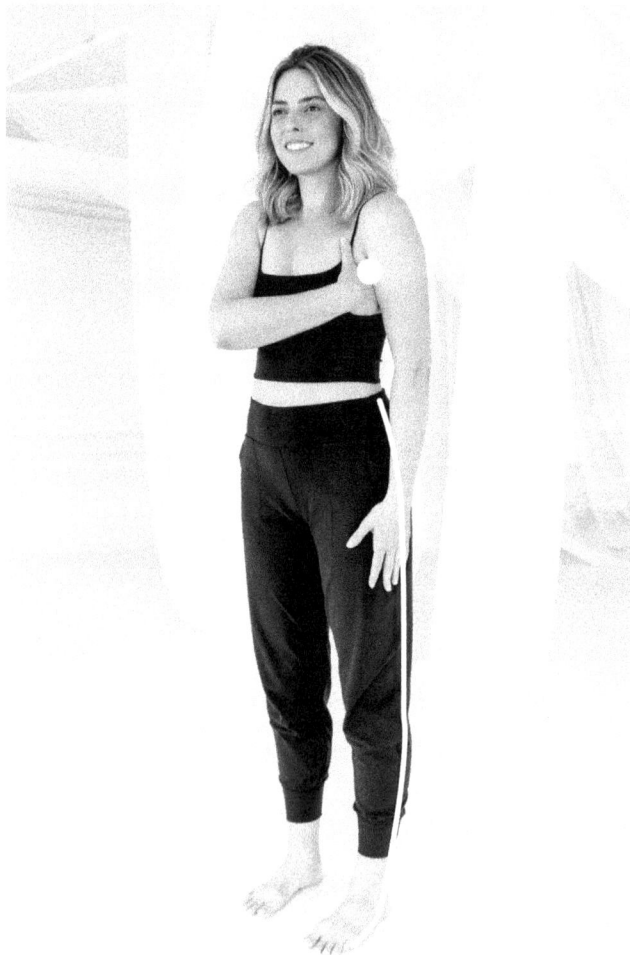

3. Hold these places for at least three to five minutes.

4. Switch sides and place your left hand under your right armpit, laying your right arm anywhere along the lateral side of your right leg.

5. Hold these places for at least three to five minutes.

Penetrating Flow

When: I would do this hold after the other ones or if I didn't have time to do all of them, I would do just this one.

Why: The penetrating flow radiant circuit is how chi is transferred from the mother to the baby at the time of birth. From there, it flows into the kidney meridian where it is then distributed to the rest of the fourteen meridians. Because it is the deepest of the radiant circuits, holding it last reinforces the work of holding the other radiant circuits and allows those shifts to move more deeply into the body.

How:

1. This is best done lying down. Place the back side of your left hand just above the back side of your left hip bone.

2. Place your right hand flat on top of your front right hip bone.

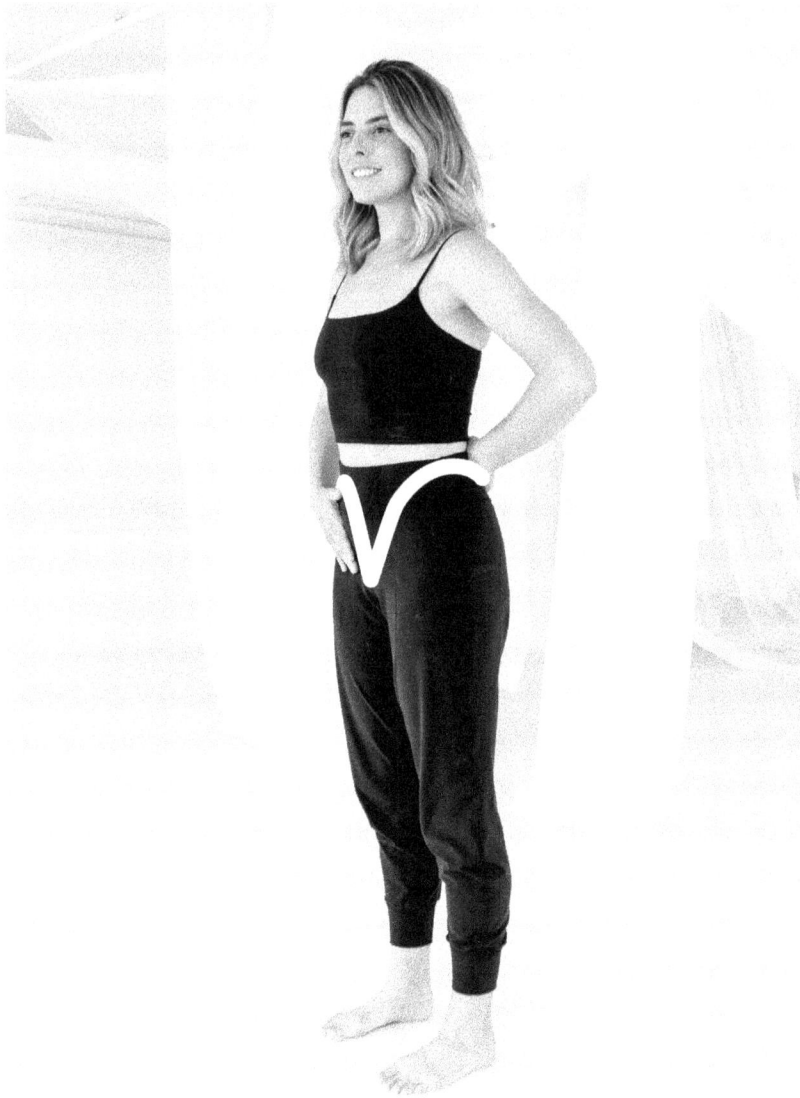

3. Hold for at least three to five minutes.

4. Switch hands so the back of your right hand is on the back of your right hip bone.

5. Place your left hand on top of your front left hip bone.

6. Hold for at least three to five minutes.

Addressing and balancing these three fundamental energy systems—triple warmer, crossover patterns and radiant circuits—were my core arsenal throughout every phase of my treatment.

Chapters 12 through 14 will focus on specific energy techniques you can use while undergoing chemotherapy, surgery, and radiation. It is not imperative to know how to energy test in order to do any of these techniques, but energy testing is a handy tool to have at your disposal. In this book, we will focus on a simple method called self-testing.

Energy Self-Testing

When: Whenever you want to learn information about your body. This technique is not intended to be used to discover other information such as: Should I buy more Apple shares? It is designed to mine the body's wisdom so as to help the body heal itself.

Why: The body holds a reservoir of energies and information. Energy testing is a biofeedback mechanism that reveals information about the body. Developing the ability to self-test is a valuable tool that can help you throughout your life.

How: The body doesn't lie. It will convey the truth if you ask it in the proper way. Using the body as a pendulum, you can discover the truth by understanding whether your body is attracted to or repelled by something.

You will need to be standing for this exercise. It's easy for your mind to get in the way of your body, so you will need to start with a "baseline" test to make sure your answers are accurate.

1. While standing, take an inhale through your nose and exhale through your mouth.
2. At the bottom of your exhale, state your name out loud: "*My name is _____.*"
3. Notice if your body moves forward or backwards after you make the statement. It should move forward if it is a true statement.
4. Now take an inhale through your nose and exhale through your mouth and state a name that is clearly not your own like: "*My name is Sponge Bob.*"
5. Your body should move backwards since this is a false statement.
6. You are now ready to ask your body a question.
7. You want to ask a question that has to do with your physical health, for example, whether a food or supplement is beneficial for you or whether an organ needs help. (Only licensed healthcare providers can energy test a medication's dosage.)
8. Place the substance or supplement on your solar plexus, located just above your navel.

9. Now using your body as a pendulum, ask it a specific question. I always ask the question at the bottom of my exhale. Keep the question simple – not too many words. Wait and see if your body moves forward or backwards in response to your question.

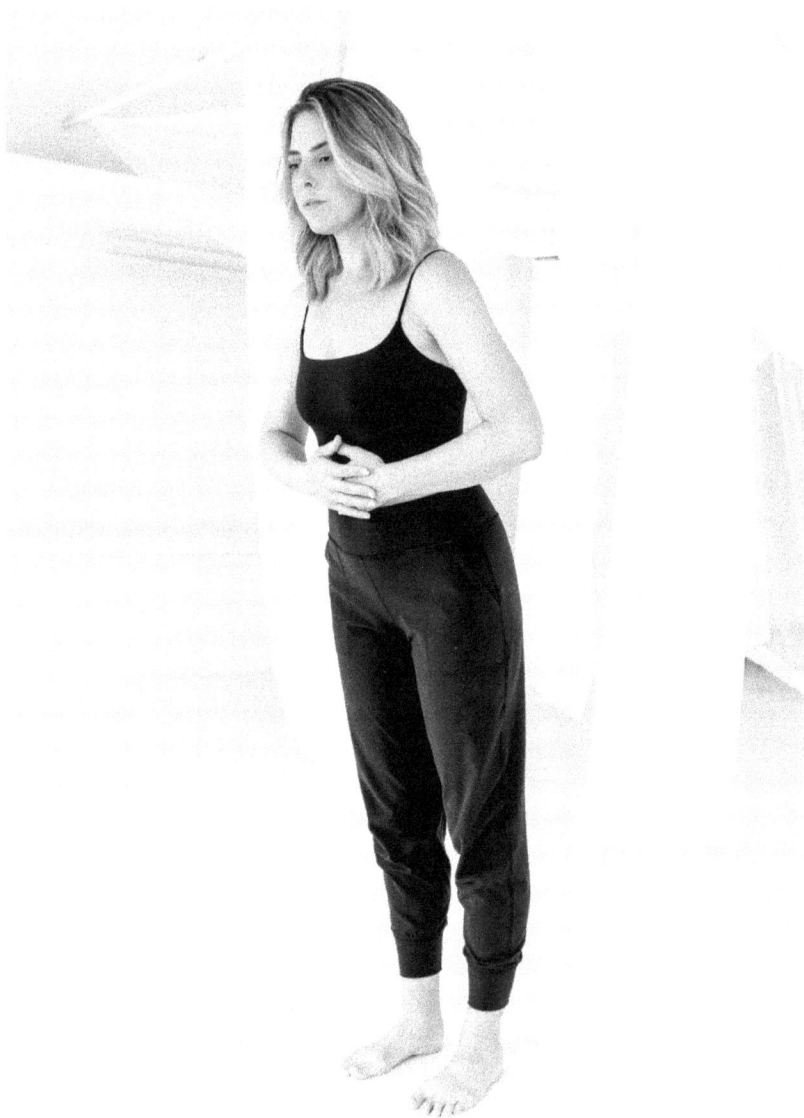

Chapter 12

Preparation and Chemotherapy

My husband was diagnosed with Stage 4 head and neck cancer in November 2018, right after Thanksgiving. We were stunned by the news, but we knew we were going to do everything we could to fight for his life. When I first met Dianne, I was immediately embraced by her warmth. She was compassionate, caring and very eager to help. It was at the lowest point in my life when I was desperate and scared. I hated feeling hopeless and not knowing what I could do to improve my husband's diagnosis. For me, life without him was not an option, so I relied heavily upon Dianne for her guidance and expertise in Eden Energy Medicine. I never thought that I would meet a healer like Dianne. At the time, I didn't know anything about Energy Medicine, but I was open-minded.

After meeting Dianne, I knew she was exactly what we needed to help us navigate our difficult journey ahead. After a deep dive into Eden Energy Medicine with Dianne, his health improved measurably. Following Dianne's suggestions for treating my husband at home also empowered me and made me feel like I could make a difference in his treatment and recovery. It was a blessing to have Dianne in our lives. I couldn't imagine what these past 5 years would have been like without her.

For the first few months, we saw her once a week. I accompanied my husband to all of his sessions so that Dianne could teach me what to do at home. After every session, my husband would tell me he felt less stressed and more relaxed.

He would start with the daily routine in the morning and before bedtime. I would spend anywhere from 60-90 minutes holding certain pressure points to relieve his pain and symptoms. During his first four rounds of chemotherapy, I would start off with nightly session of the Brazilian Toe Hold. Dianne told me it would help with any nausea and side effects from his chemo. Sure enough, he never got any serious side effects from his chemo sessions. No nausea or vomiting, not even a loss of appetite. He was mentally and physically strong and determined to fight.

Dianne provided us with the tools and shared her expertise in Eden Energy Medicine which helped reduce the negative side effects of his treatment. Both of us benefited emotionally from her guidance in coping with his diagnosis.

My husband has been in remission for almost 5 years now and I am still using Eden Energy Medicine for maintenance. From doing Figure 8s to clearing his chakras, using the Neurovasculars, calming triple warmer, working with the electrics, the daily routine and the Brazilian Toe Hold and many more protocols — all of them helped my husband emotionally and physically. I strongly believe that Dianne and Eden Energy Medicine made the difference in my husband's recovery process. From the bottom of my heart, I have so much gratitude and love for Dianne. She gave us hope and healing when we needed it most. She changed our lives for the better.

Elaine F.

Most people with a cancer diagnosis discover fairly quickly, it's not just the cancer treatment that is time-consuming, exhausting, expensive, and depressing; it's also all the preliminary testing, biopsies, MRIs, CT scans, echocardiograms, labs, and other appointments that begin to consume one's life. Prior to a scan, procedure, or test, I had lots of energy medicine tools to use, but I also developed some energy hacks to keep my radiant circuit energies flowing. Something as simple as having a book I loved to read and reading it only when I was in the waiting room would keep my body in positive anticipation of reading the book instead of feeling anxious about the procedure. I would choose books that were meditative or energy based so I could use the technique I was reading about while on the table.

For example, I would enter into a meditative state while undergoing an MRI and imagine the noise of the machine tapping away the cancer cells, or I would surround myself with a color that represented peace and health while having a procedure done. When I was really miserable undergoing chemo, I would go to Instagram and watch only beautiful things. If I was feeling nauseous or having other side effects, I would watch scenes of Switzerland, birds or horses to keep my mind in a happy and peaceful place. This really helped counteract whatever unpleasant scenario I might be facing.

The following are some of the EEM techniques I used to prepare my body for the tests, procedures, and treatments.

Temporal Tapping

When: I started this technique several days prior to a test, procedure, or treatment to prepare my body for what was to come and help prevent it from going into stress response.

Why: Because the brain's limbic system is in the driver's seat when we encounter stress, we tend to get stuck in a negative, repetitive feedback loop. By tapping on both sides of the brain, you are simultaneously directing triple warmer and balancing the right and left hemispheres. By tapping backwards on the triple warmer meridian, you are taking energy out of the meridian and calming your body's stress response. Your triple warmer will follow because you are giving it explicit direction. It helps to involve as many senses as possible, so the message penetrates the nervous system. This technique is super simple, and it works great. It can be used to achieve any goal.

How: Begin by making a goal: What is it you want to achieve? Or, put another way, what do you want to avoid? For example, if you have a fear of needles, your goal might be: *I want to have blood drawn without feeling nauseous or faint.*

1. Choose two statements that reflect your goal. Both affirmations need to be positive, but one must have a negative word in it. The right side of the brain is the more creative hemisphere, so using a purely positive affirmation on that side will be easily accepted by the right half. The left side of the brain is the more critical side, so by tapping in a statement that has a negative word in it, you "trick" the left side into accepting the goal.

    Using our needles example, a statement for the right side might be:
    It's easy for me to have blood drawn.

    The statement for the left side might be:
    I have no fear of needles.

Be sure both statements are positive even though the one on the left side has a negative word in it.

2. You will be tapping these statements backwards along the triple warmer meridian.

3. Start with the left hand on the left side of your head.

4. Starting at the temple, tap behind the ear while saying the statement five times out loud.

5. It's important to say the affirmations so both the mind and body can hear them.

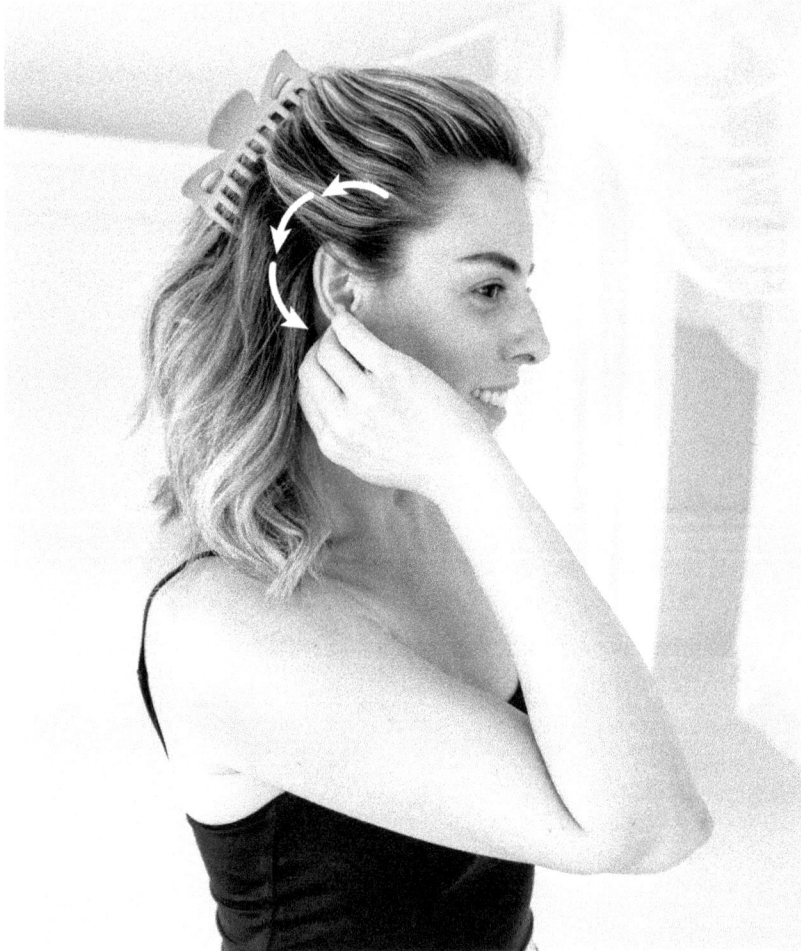

6. You can energy test to find out how many times a day you need to do the exercise in order for your body to begin to believe it and act accordingly, but a general rule of

thumb is to do it four or five times a day and/or whenever the stressor you are address-ing triggers you. Try to connect it to a daily activity, like eating, so you remember to do it.

7. If you were raised speaking another language, use that language when you do the tapping. That way, it will penetrate better into your subconscious mind.

Substance Repatterning

When: I used this technique to help prepare my body to receive the chemotherapy infusions.

Why: By doing something as simple as writing on a piece of paper the words of the med-ications you will be receiving and placing that in your pocket, the vibration of the words can start to penetrate your energy field and your body will start to come into resonance with that frequency. This, in turn, will allow your triple warmer to be less reactive and more accommodat-ing to the medication. Combined with temporal tapping, this technique allowed my body to be more accepting of the toxic medications it was receiving. One time, I didn't know I was going to receive an on-body injector of Neulasta at the end of my chemo treatment, and my body reacted to that worse than the chemo! I learned after that to be sure to get a list of every medication or procedure I was going to receive prior to my treatment so my body wouldn't have any surprises.

How: Several days before your infusion, take a small piece of paper and write the names of the medications and/or procedures you are going to be receiving on it. Include every medica-tion, even if it is a steroid or noncancer drug. Use a separate piece of paper for each medication, test, or procedure. Put the folded pieces of paper in the pocket of what you are wearing that day. Do this every day, including the day you receive your infusion.

While Undergoing Chemotherapy

Acupressure Toe Hold

You will need a partner for this.

When: This technique should be done while you are undergoing chemotherapy or shortly thereafter. Ideally, it would be done while the most toxic drugs are being infused.

Why: Each toe and finger is the beginning or endpoint of a meridian. Holding these points activates chi and releases stuck energy in the meridians by creating a circuit of energy between the practitioner's hands and the recipient's feet. Holding for at least three minutes allows the energy to circulate throughout all fourteen meridians.

A clinical study was conducted using this protocol at the Dana-Farber Cancer Institute in Boston, Massachusetts. Seventy-five breast cancer patients received this treatment while undergoing their chemotherapy infusion. One hundred percent reported less pain, nausea, anxiety, and neuropathy as a result of the treatment.[16]

How: Your feet will need to be elevated during this procedure. Most chemotherapy centers have chairs that can elevate your feet. Your partner will need to be sitting in a chair that allows them to access your feet and still be comfortable. It's important that both of you are comfortable because once your partner begins holding your toes, they should not sever the connection until the protocol is complete. You can be barefoot or keep your socks on.

To prepare:

You and your partner should be well-hydrated, and the practioner should first open their hand and your foot gaits.

Opening the Hand and Foot Gaits

1. Open your right palm and with your left thumb, massage from the base of the right hand across the palm to each finger.
2. Moving to the little finger, continue to massage up the finger until you get to the tip.
3. Pull the energy off the little finger.
4. Move back to the base of the palm. Massage up the ring finger.

5. Take the energy off the ring finger.
6. Continue to do this with the rest of the fingers.
7. Do a couple of passes to allow stuck energy to leave the body.
8. Turn the hand over and massage from the base of the hand at the wrist and move up to each finger.
9. Pull the energy off each fingertip.
10. Do a couple of passes to allow the stuck energy to leave the body.
11. Switch and do the left hand.

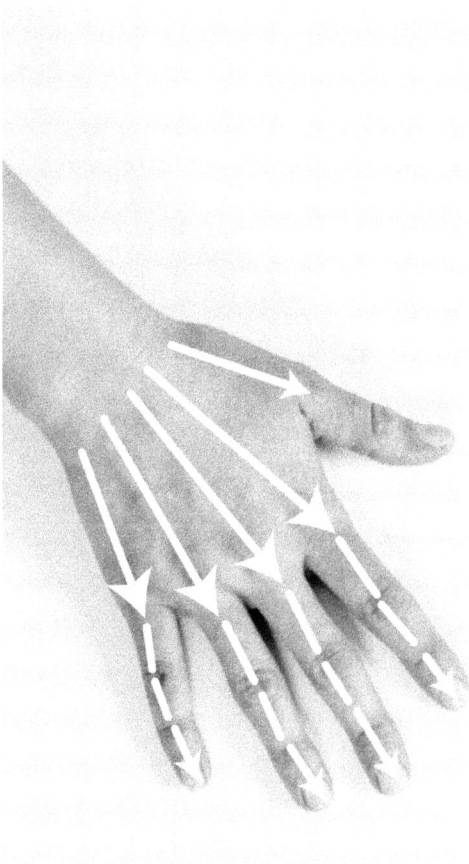

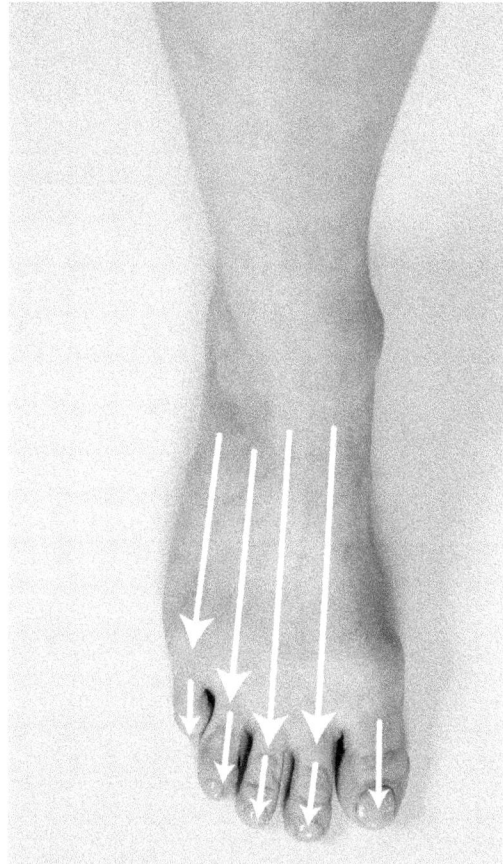

12. Your partner should do the same massage on your feet, starting at the ankles and moving down in between the metatarsal bones, out to the toes, pulling the energy off each toe.

13. Do a couple of passes to allow the stuck energy to leave the body.

14. Moving to the bottom of the feet, they should press deeply as they move up the foot towards the toes. Pull the energy off each toe.

15. Do a couple of passes to allow the stuck energy to leave the body.

Protocol: Written from the caregiver's perspective

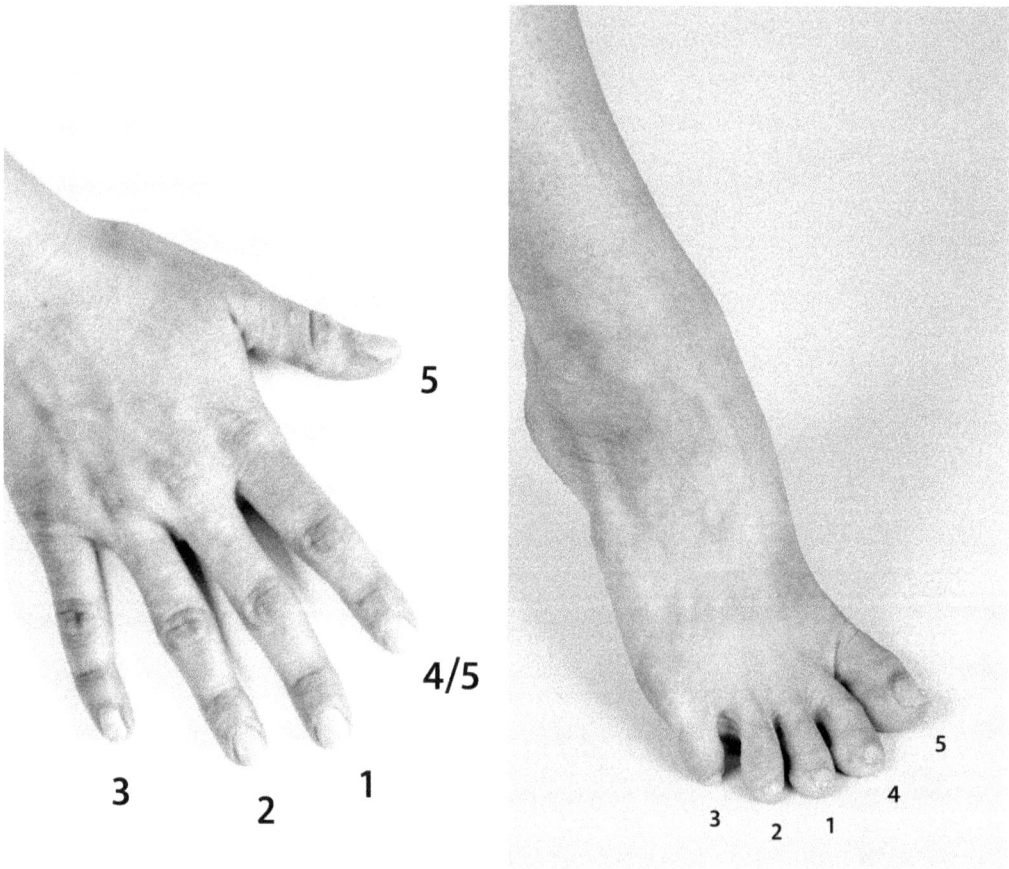

As you move from toe to toe, do not lose touch with the recipient's feet. This is important in order to keep the energy circuit flowing between you.

1. Facing the recipient, place both of your thumbs underneath their third toes.

2. Place your third fingers on top of the recipient's third toes at the nail beds.

3. Hold with some pressure so there is contact between you but not so much as to constrict blood flow.

4. Hold for three to five minutes or until you sense the need to move on. If you are able to feel energy, move once you feel a synchronized pulse between the toes.

5. While keeping your third fingers on top of the recipient's third toes, slide your thumb over to the bottom of the recipient's fourth toes.

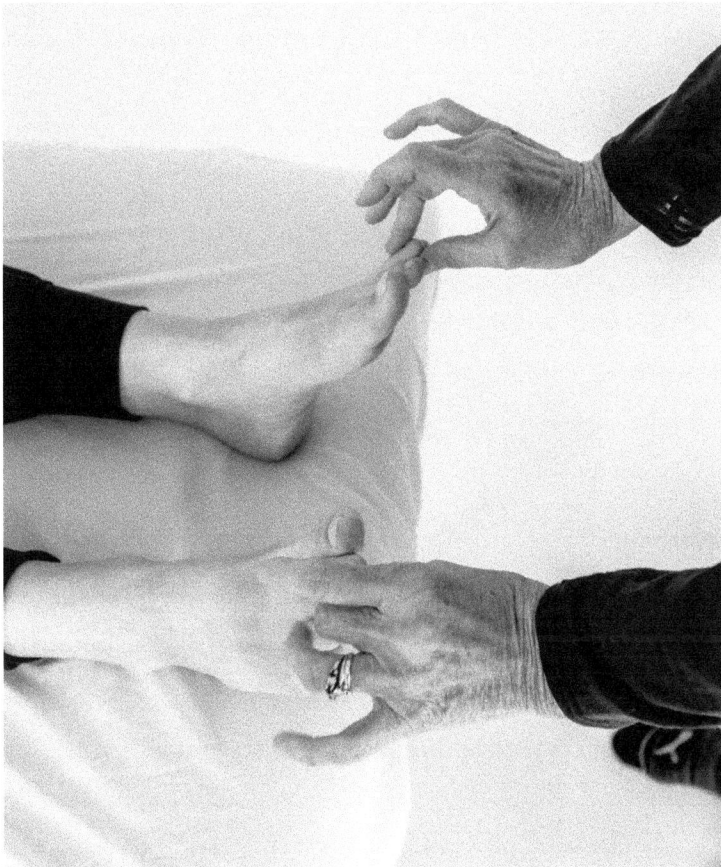

6. Let go of your third fingers on the third toes and place your fourth fingers on top of their fourth toes.

7. Hold for three to five minutes.

8. Keeping your fourth fingers on top of their fourth toes, slide both thumbs onto the bottom of their fifth toes.

9. Release your fourth fingers from the fourth toes and move your fifth fingers on top of their fifth toes.

10. Hold for three to five minutes.

11. Keeping your fifth fingers on top of their fifth toes, slide your thumbs to the bottom of their second toes.

12. Move your second fingers onto their second toes.

13. Hold for three to five minutes.

14. Keeping your second fingers on top of their second toes, slide your thumbs under their big toes.

15. Release your fingers from the second toe and place your first and second fingers onto the base corners of their big toenail beds.

16. Hold for three to five minutes.

17. End the session by pressing into the center of the ball of the foot. This is the first point on kidney meridian. Hold this point for a minute or gently pulse into the point while synchronizing your pulsing with the recipient's inhales for three breaths. This helps to further calm the nervous system and release toxins.

Chakra Preparation

You will need a partner for this.

When: Ideally, this protocol would be done while undergoing a chemotherapy infusion, but if that is not possible, it can be done afterwards. It should also be done periodically while undergoing cancer treatment as many procedures and tests interfere with your biofield and can disturb your chakras.

Why: Our biofield extends from our body outward in a 360-degree circle, essentially from your body to your fingertips. It functions as a protective layer, similar to the earth's atmosphere. Medical science views our skin as our immune system's first line of protection, but EEM sees the biofield as our body's first line of defense: the stronger the biofield, the healthier the body. Chakras sit inside the biofield and have the important job of extracting information from the environment and communicating that information into our body via the endocrine system. EEM focuses on the seven main chakras: root, womb, solar plexus, heart, throat, third eye, and crown.

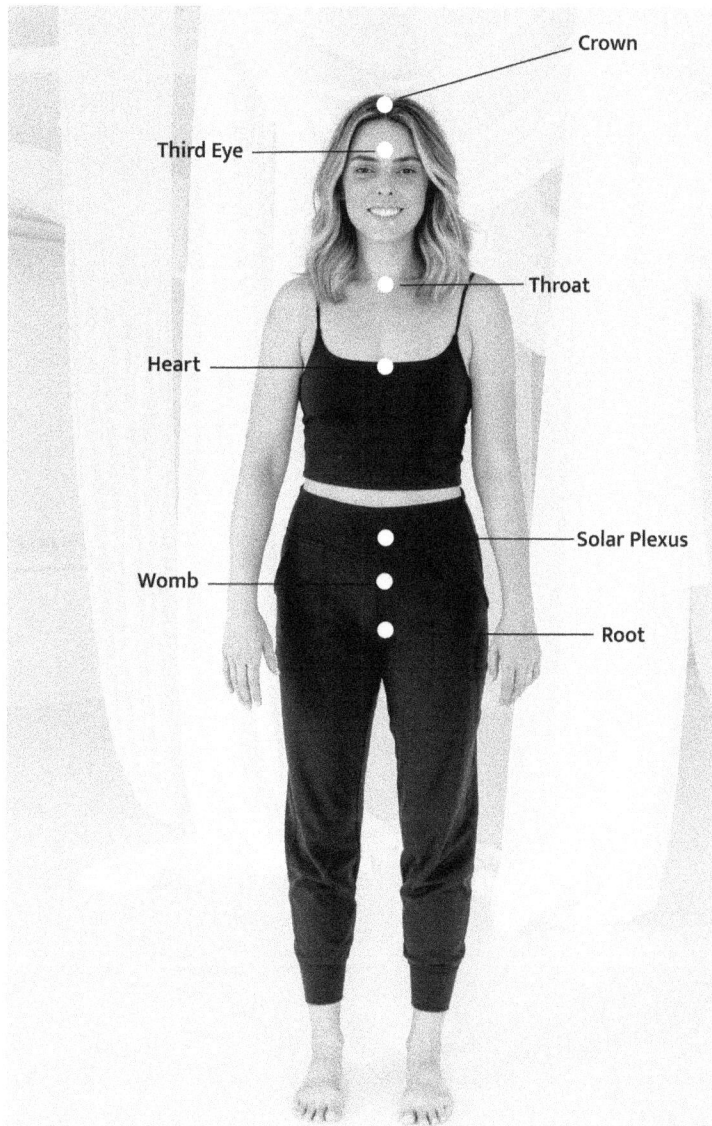

In addition to the seven main chakras, there are seven layers within each chakra. Each layer can move in a different direction, depending upon what that particular chakra is processing. You don't need to know in which direction a particular level is moving; the body will adjust to what shifts it needs to make happen. Making counterclockwise circles helps to clear toxins out of a chakra. Making clockwise circles seals in changes you have made and strengthens the chakras. The best analogy I can think of is a screw: Turning it to the left opens it up; turning it to the right locks it in place. You will want to spend several minutes making counterclockwise directions to clear the body and field of toxins, followed by a minute of a clockwise pattern at the end to seal in the clearing you have made.

VERY IMPORTANT: Never make clockwise circles over the area of a tumor regardless of where it sits in relation to a chakra. For example, in the case of someone with breast cancer, the closest chakra is the heart chakra. In that case, do not end the chakra clearing with clockwise circles, simply do the counterclockwise direction.

When we walk barefoot on the earth, energy centers and meridians in our feet absorb the environmental energy and move it up into the body. Because very few people walk barefoot today, we lose the benefits of this energy transference. Therefore, before I clear or strengthen chakras, I typically start with something called a *Vortex Revival*. This technique is essentially the same as working with the chakras, however, the vortex we are creating moves only in a counterclockwise direction. Doing this technique recreates the earth's energetic flow and also helps tap into the root chakra.

Vortex Revival

You will need a partner for this.

How: Lie down or at least have your feet elevated. Your partner can be seated initially, but eventually they will be standing up.

Protocol: Written from the caregiver's perspective

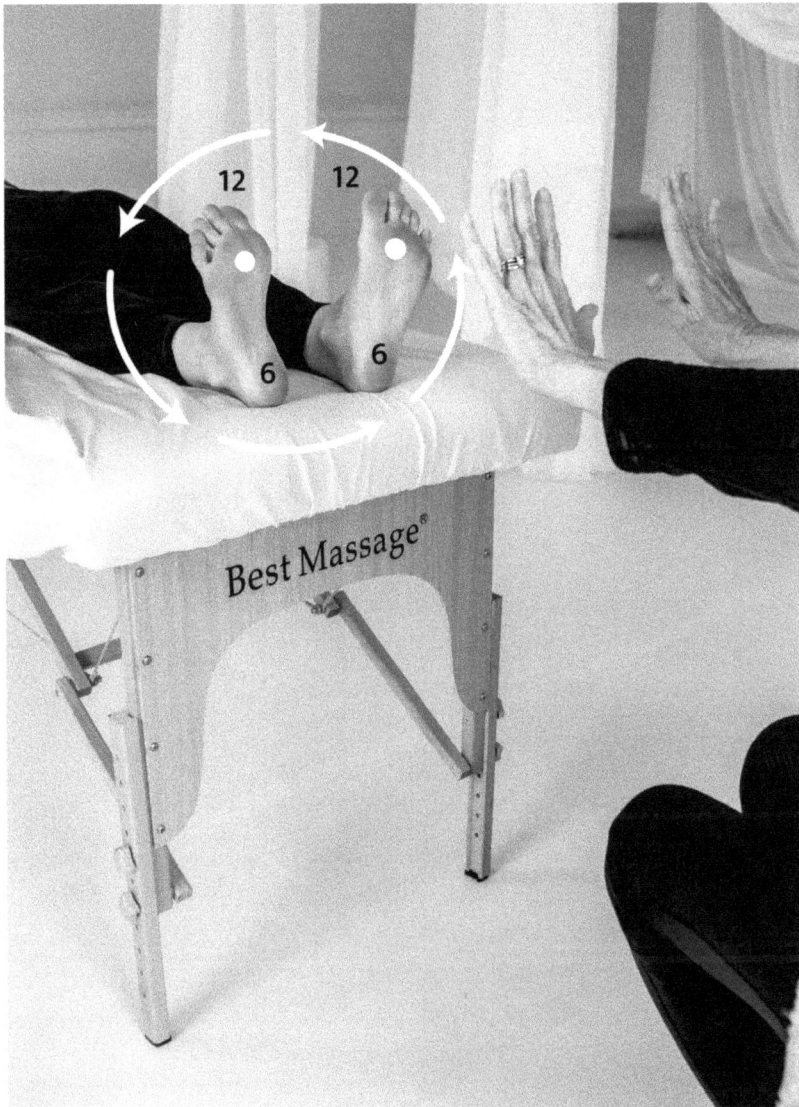

1. Stand or sit at least 18 inches away (if possible) from the recipient's feet in line with the ball of their foot.
2. Imagine there is a clock on the bottom of their feet. The 12 is located at the toes, and the 6 is at the heel.
3. Begin slowly making counterclockwise circles in line with the ball of the foot.
4. Do this for several minutes, slowly moving towards the body so you end at the feet.

Chakra Protocol

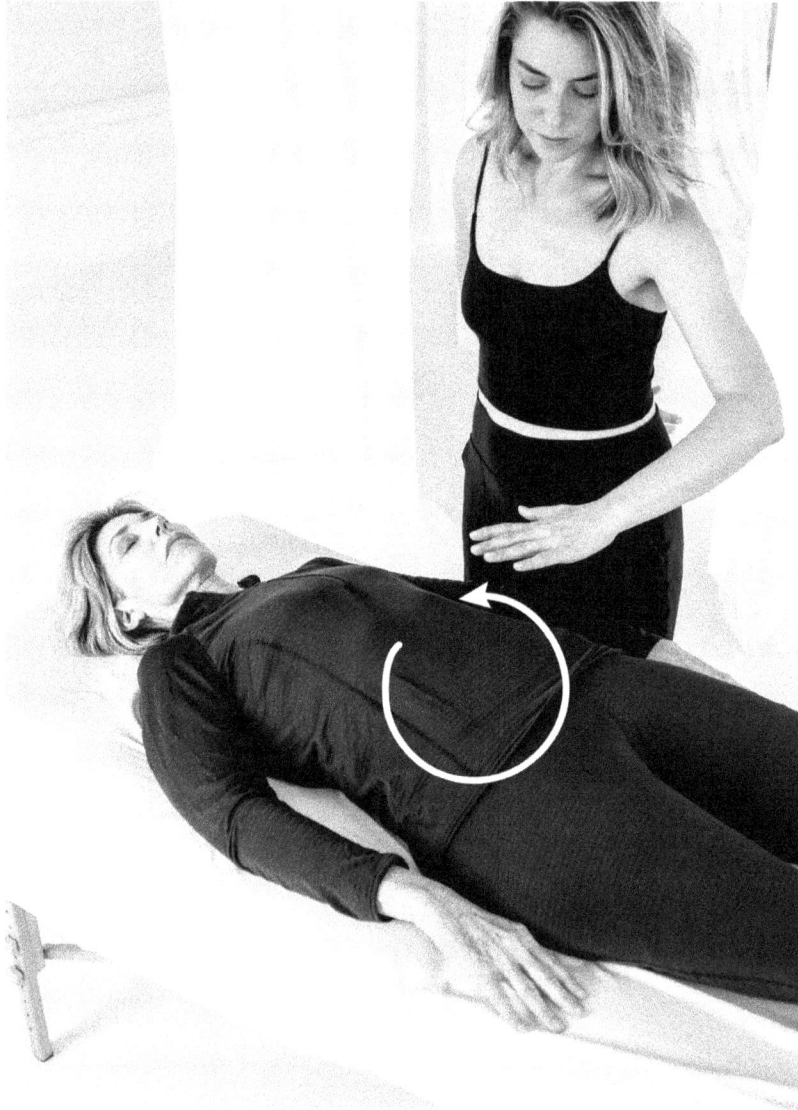

1. Move up to the first chakra located in line with the pubic bone.
2. Imagine there is a clock superimposed on the body. The 12 is in the direction of the head, and the 6 is located at the feet.

3. Flip your hand back and forth for about 30 seconds. This balances the polarity in the root chakra, which, if reversed or frozen, can lock other chakras up the line.

4. Make counterclockwise circles very slowly for several minutes about four inches off the body in line with the pubic bone.

5. End with making clockwise circles for about 30 seconds.

6. Move up the body to each chakra and do the same thing, making counterclockwise circles for several minutes and then clockwise circles for about one minute. (The exception to this rule is if you are working on a man, at the seventh chakra, start with a clockwise direction and end with a counterclockwise movement. Also, if someone is prone to headaches, start from the crown chakra and move down the body.)

If you don't have time to do a full chakra clearing, you can also 'comb' the biofield to remove toxins from the field. Starting at the head and extending out into the field, the practitioner would slowly move their hands down your body and off your feet. They should do this for several minutes, making passes from your head to your feet and end by shaking the energy off their hands.

Dealing with Side Effects

This list is not exhaustive and addresses only the most common side effects experienced during chemotherapy.

Nausea

Fortunately, today there are medications like Zofran and Compazine that counteract nausea well without too many side effects. If they aren't working for you or you want a more energetic approach, there are several techniques you can use.

Massaging Stomach 36

Why: Perhaps the most famous point in TCM, Stomach 36 is known as the "three-mile point" because Chinese warriors discovered they could walk further if they massaged this point. Massaging Stomach 36 can help address any abdominal issue, including nausea.

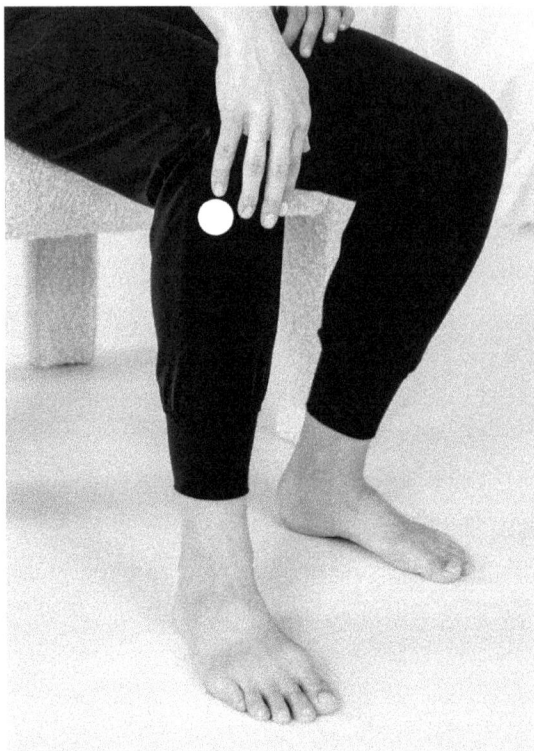

How:

1. Begin by sitting on a chair.
2. Place your palm on your bent knee. The space where your little finger lands, in between your kneecap and your tibia, is where the point is located. For many people, this point will be tender, so it can be relatively easy to find. If you have trouble finding the point exactly, put two fingers in the muscles between the tibia and fibula, and you will be in the correct place.
3. Massage deeply for a minute or two.
4. You can also just hold the space with the intention to relax the meridian or tap or pulse the point.
5. Adding an essential oil like lavender or peppermint to the point can also help.

6. Do both right and left legs a few times a day. You cannot "overdo" massaging the point, but don't do it so much as to bruise yourself.

Tapping or Holding Stomach 1

Why: The stomach meridian starts just below the eye and ends at the second toe. The meridian governs the organ, so tapping the meridian will send a signal from the meridian to the organ to relax and regulate. Holding lightly or tapping this point will help send energy to the stomach and calm it.

How:
1. Find the highest point on your cheekbone in line with your pupil.
2. Tap lightly for a minute.
3.   Place one finger lightly on the point and place your other hand gently across your forehead for several minutes.
4. Switch hands, tap the other cheekbone, then hold the stomach point while placing your other palm on your forehead.

Holding or Tapping Stomach Meridian Beginning and Endpoints

Why: Sometimes you are too sick to do much of anything, but something as simple as holding or tapping a meridian's beginning or end points will create a circuit of energy that can free up blocked energy in a meridian. Balancing the meridian will, in turn, balance the organ and can help ease your suffering.

How:
1. Hold both the beginning and endpoints simultaneously. Stomach 1 is located on the highest point of the cheekbone. Stomach 45 is located at the lateral side of the second toenail (towards the third toe).
2. Hold these points for several minutes.
3. You can also hold, tap or spin a cut-glass crystal on these points. (The cut-glass crystals can be found on Amazon under Suncatchers or you can make them yourself.)

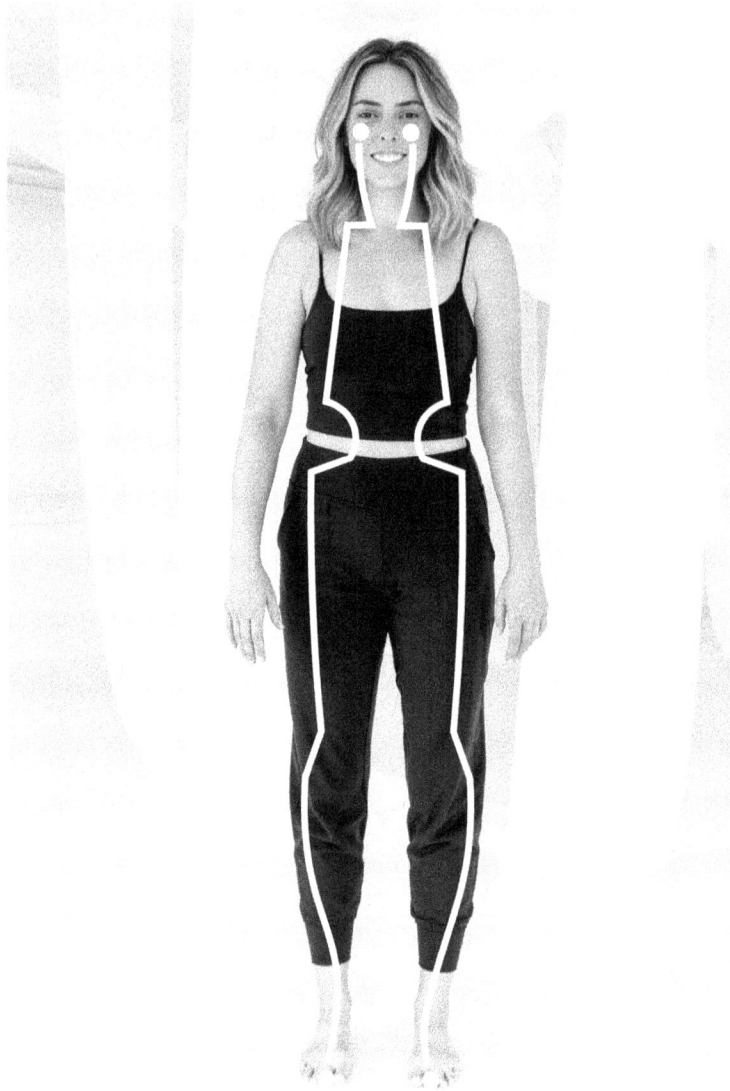

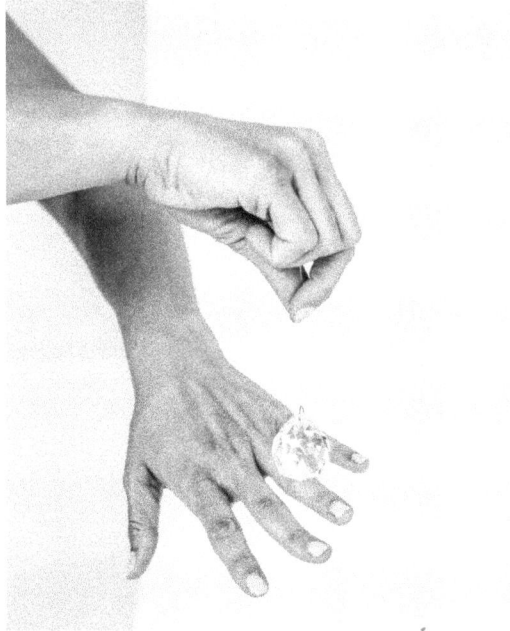

Alopecia

Hair loss isn't as inevitable as it once was with chemotherapy treatment. There is something called a *cooling cap* that essentially freezes your scalp while the chemotherapy is being infused. There is no guarantee that your hair won't fall out at all, but it definitely slows down the process. And it's a painful process, I might add. So, there is the pain of hair loss and the flip side of waiting for your hair to grow back. This exercise can help with both.

Crown Pull

Why: Stimulating the scalp accomplishes several things:
- It encourages stuck chi to move out of the head, where many meridian pathways run.
- It helps move the cerebral spinal fluid along its pathway.
- It helps open up the suture lines, which can move ever so slightly or get jammed.
- It helps stimulate hair follicles to produce more hair growth.

I found doing this exercise helped both with decreasing the pain I experienced while losing my hair and with increasing the thickness and pace at which my new hair grew in. (It's also great for headaches!)

How: You will be massaging from the forehead to the hairline, then to the back of the head, one finger's width at a time.

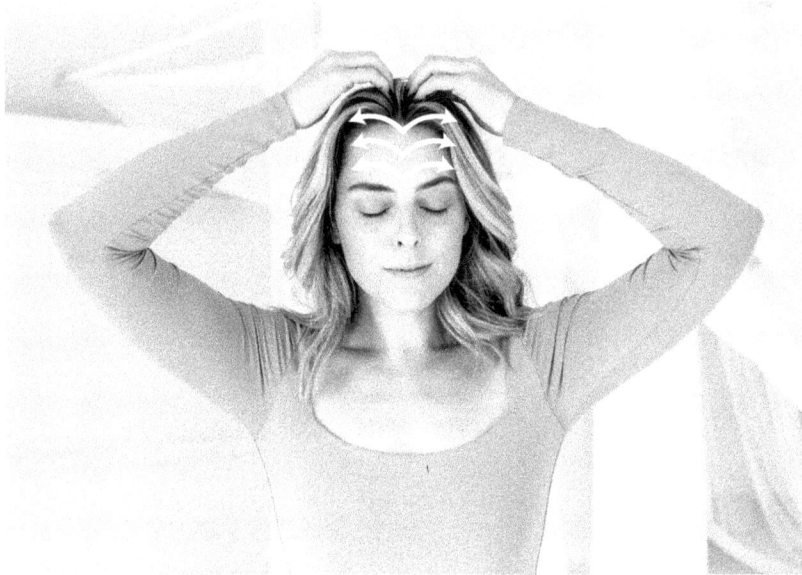

1. Start by placing your fingertips at the center of your forehead.
2. Push in with a bit of pressure and pull your fingers out to your temple.
3. Move your fingers one finger's width up from the center of your forehead and do the same motion again, pressing in on the forehead and pulling out to the sides.
4. Move up another finger's width. This time you will be at the hairline. Do the same motion again.
5. Continue to do this pushing in and pulling out movement up through your scalp, across the top and back of your head, ending at the neckline.
6. Make another three or four passes from your forehead to your occipital ridge (where you skull and neck meet).
7. Do this at least twice a day.

Constipation

Most of my chemotherapy agents caused diarrhea, but some of the antinausea or pain medications can cause constipation. I found two things that helped me when I suffered from constipation. The first was to change my diet. I began every day with a green smoothie consisting of kale, spinach or other greens, flax seed, and frozen fruit. In addition, I worked my large intestine *neurolymphatic points*. These are reflex points that run along the lateral sides (outside) of the legs between the hips and the knees.

Massaging Large Intestine Neurolymphatics

Why: Neurolymphatic reflex points exist throughout the body and correspond to each organ and meridian. The lymphatic system doesn't have a pump, so massaging these points acts like a switch to turn on the lymphatic channels for that particular organ. Our large intestine must continually process food, toxins, bacteria, medications, and waste products. Massaging the large intestine neurolymphatic points regularly helps clear these toxins from our body. The right leg from the knee to the hip bone corresponds to the ascending colon; the left leg from the hip to the knee corresponds to the descending colon. Massaging these points can also provide relief for lower back or hip pain.

How: This exercise can be done lying down, sitting, or standing. I found it was easiest to access these points by lying on my side, especially if I was feeling weak or tired. Someone can also do this for you.

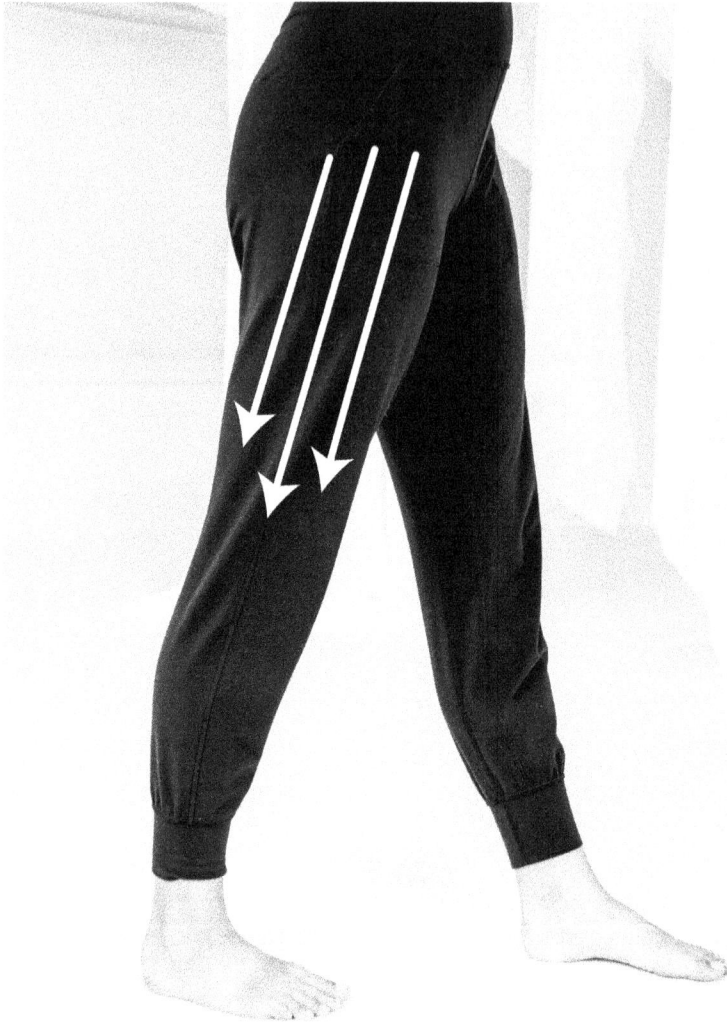

1. Start by lightly massaging your leg along the sides of your body from your hip bone to your knee (essentially the iliotibial band—IT band). It is a fairly wide area, so don't miss any spaces. Do this for a minute or two.
2. Once you have softened the muscles, start pressing more deeply to see if there are any tender areas. Make note of those areas.
3. Come back to the hip. Slowly move down the leg to the tender areas one by one

spending some time massaging each of these points. You want to put pressure on them, but not so much as to bruise yourself. On a scale of 0 to 10, you want your pain tolerance to be between a 5-to-7 pressure, painful but not excruciating. Not putting enough pressure will make it ineffective.

4. Slowly move down the leg until you get to your knee, massaging each tender point.

5. Go back to the hip and massage again. Notice if the area that was tender before becomes less so. Continue doing this for another few minutes. Typically, when you revisit the points that were initially tender, they will be less so the second time you massage. This means that the inflammation has started to dissipate. In some cases, you might find the leg becomes more tender. This usually means that the inflammation was being masked by the superficial muscles and, over time, is starting to reveal itself.

6. Switch to your left leg. You may notice as you get towards the left knee, it becomes more tender. This area of the leg corresponds to the rectum, so if you are suffering from constipation, it may be the most tender here. Spending more time here can help facilitate better bowel movements.

7. Be sure to drink lots of water after doing this work because you are encouraging the release of toxins and you want to flush them out of your system.

8. If you feel nauseous at any point, stop immediately and do the *neurovascular hold* for several minutes.

9. Sometimes, particularly with chemotherapy treatment, there are so many toxins in the body, releasing them can be too much too soon. Slow down in this case and only do a little bit a day.

10. Do this daily if you are suffering from constipation. Otherwise, try to do it at least once a week to help rid your body of toxins.

Diarrhea

Many chemotherapy agents cause diarrhea because they target rapidly dividing cells and our intestinal lining consists of rapidly dividing cells. At first, diarrhea was the worst side effect for me, but I was able to get a handle on it by drinking kefir and later by taking calcium bentonite clay. I used *Medi-Clay FX* from Premier Research Labs, and it was a game changer. I would take a capsule as soon as I had a sign of trouble, and it would settle my intestines down so I might have a loose stool, but no diarrhea. You have to be careful with this product if you are using it for diarrhea. If you take too much, it can cause constipation, so you want to monitor how your body responds to it. Massaging the neurolymphatics can also help.

Massaging Large Intestine Neurolymphatics

This is the same technique as for constipation, but instead of massaging downwards from the hips to the knees, you would massage upwards from the knees towards the hips. This can help slow down peristalsis (the movement of food along the intestinal tract) and begin to reduce inflammation in the colon.

Mouth Sores

What was one of the worst side effects from Day One of treatment proved to be the easiest to fix: Sucking on ice chips while getting my infusion. The technical term is *cryotherapy*, and it works like a charm. If you do get mouth sores, oil pulling can be helpful. Oil pulling is an ancient Ayurvadic practice that uses oil like mouthwash. Swishing the oil for several minutes can help heal the tender tissue in and around the mouth. When finished, spit it out. I used organic coconut oil.

Neuropathy

Dealing with neuropathy is not obvious because it can become a chronic problem or become exacerbated not just by chemotherapy but also immunotherapy and even radiation. It can come on after treatment and its impact can be cumulative, so you might not realize you have it until after you are finished. In fact, neuropathy is probably my only late effect. In fact, neuropathy was one of my only late effects. Fortunately, it resolved, but I didn't have someone available to do the acupressure toe hold for me every time I was getting an infusion, and it wasn't until my last chemotherapy session that I learned icing one's feet and hands can prevent neuropathy. Amazon sells cold therapy gloves and socks you can wear during your infusions. You can also ask the nursing staff to give you ice packs to place on your feet and hands during your infusions. Taking vitamin B-12 and alpha-lipoic acid is known to help, but there are also several energy medicine interventions you can use.

Acupressure Toe Hold

This technique is described in detail under *Preparing for Chemotherapy* (See Page 128). If you use cold therapy packs, use those during the most toxic part of your infusion and do the toe hold treatment before or after that. Your partner can also do this treatment for you at home to encourage your body to release toxins after your infusions. When working with my cancer clients, I would have their loved one perform this treatment several times a week.

Opening the Gaits

This is one of the preparatory steps for the *Acupressure Toe Hold* (See Page 128), but it can be done independently of the treatment and is particularly good for neuropathy. Try to do it at least twice a day. Combining it with a relaxing Epsom salt, baking soda, or essential oil-infused foot bath can also help facilitate the removal of toxins from the body.

Spinning a Crystal at the Fingers and Toes Endpoints

Spinning a crystal for about thirty seconds on each finger and toe can help balance the meridians, calm the nervous system, and move toxins out of the body. Do this regularly, particularly after you have had an infusion or are taking toxic medications. (See Page 140-141.)

Spooning the Feet

When: Do at least once daily.

Why: Every cell in our body is like a small battery with a negative and positive charge. This polarity expands to every muscle, tissue, and organ. Healers like Donna Eden and Tom Tam believe that dysfunction in the electrical aspect of the body is at the root of many illnesses, including cancer. The earth also has polarity; namely, the North and South Poles. Historically, people lived closer to the earth and exchanged energies with it by walking barefoot or setting their schedules in harmony with nature. Today, we drive cars, stay up late at night, and walk with shoes on concrete pavements. The energies we formerly exchanged with the earth that kept our polarity in balance are no longer absorbed by the body through the feet. In addition, toxins, environmental interferences like Wi-Fi, and medical procedures can reverse the body's natural polarity. This, in turn, can have a negative impact on our health. Since we won't be going back to walking barefoot anytime soon, we can restore the natural polarity in our body by doing something as simple as smoothing a stainless-steel spoon on the soles of our feet. I have a spoon next to my bed and spoon my feet every night. It can also help you to sleep better!

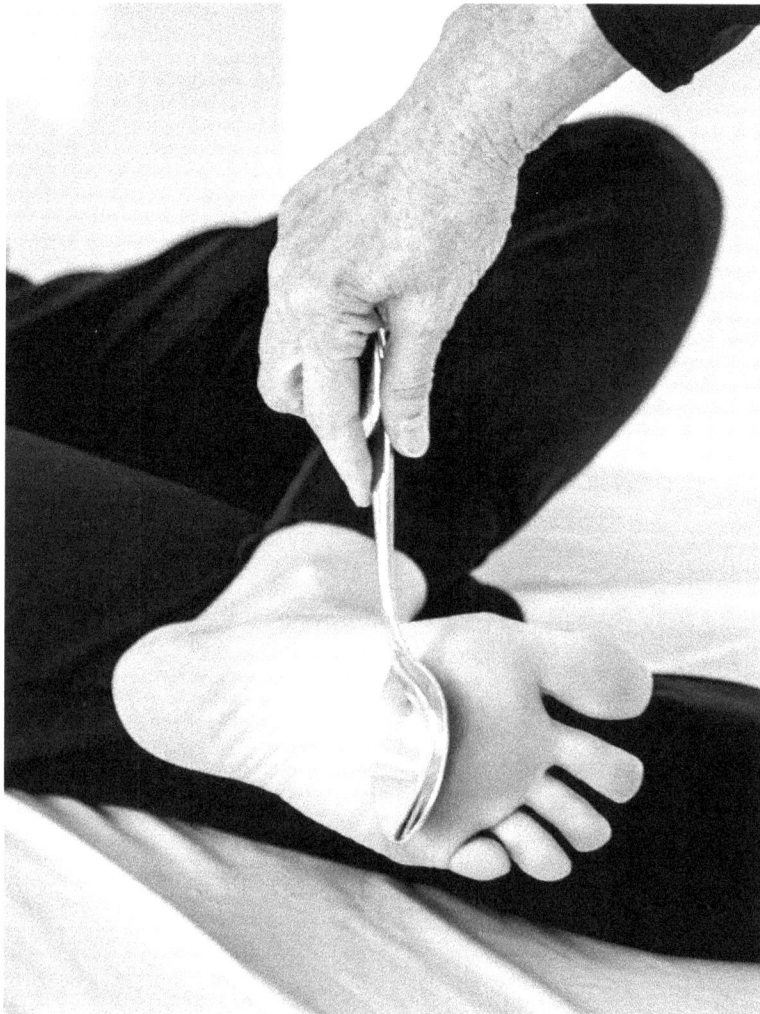

How:

1. Find a spoon that has a magnetic quality to it (it will attract a magnet).
2. Use the back side of the spoon to smooth the soles of your feet. It doesn't matter in which manner you start or finish; just be sure to cover every portion of your foot, from the toes to the heels.
3. Make about 30 passes on each foot.

Bone or Joint Pain

Word on the street (Facebook cancer groups) is that over-the-counter allergy medications like Claritin or Zyrtec can help prevent bone pain. Acupuncture, yoga, and massage can also help. I did all those things along with EEM, and I experienced significant joint and bone pain only once.

Connecting Heaven and Earth

When: This can be done daily, but if joint pain is an issue, it should be done several times throught the day.

Why: The chi in our body tends to get stuck in the joints. Opening up the joints or the space between the bones (the gaits) can help keep the chi flowing through the body. EEM teaches that pain is blocked energy and energy needs space to move, so moving that space can alleviate pain. Even prior to my cancer diagnosis, this exercise helped tremendously with the joint pain I experienced from rheumatoid arthritis.

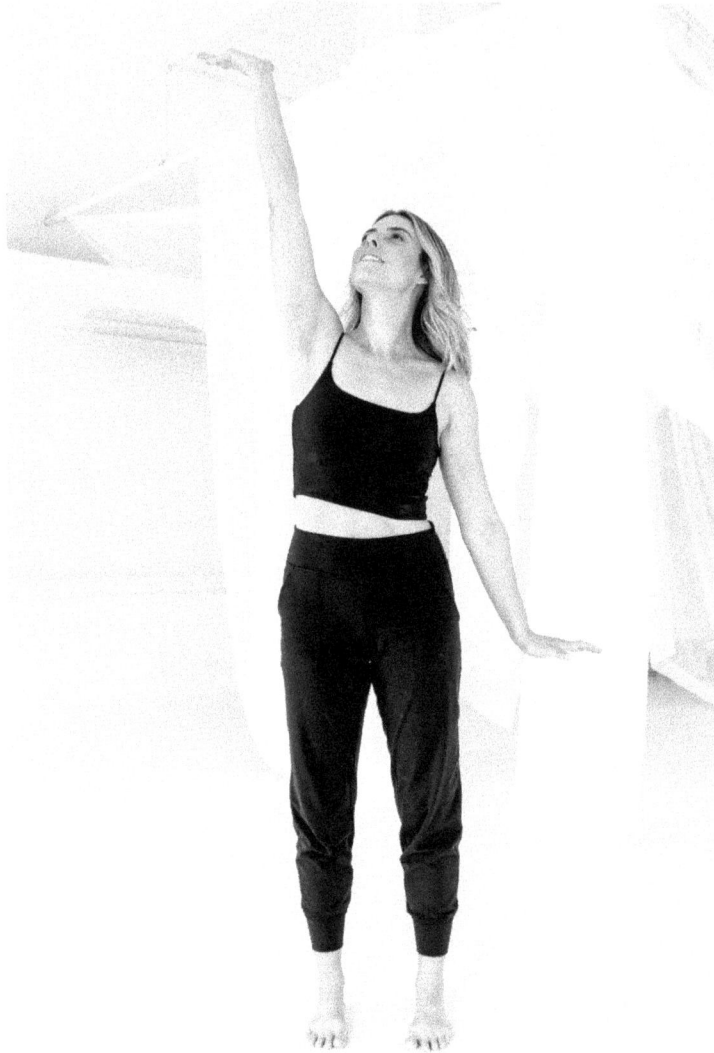

How: Ideally, this would be done standing, but if you cannot stand, it can be done sitting down.

1. Place your hands on your thighs.
2. Inhale and place your hands at your heart in a prayerful position.
3. Exhale and extend your arms away from your body in opposite directions with one arm reaching above your head and the other arm reaching down to the ground.

4. Flatten your palms so they are perpendicular to your body.

5. Inhale and look up at the palm above your head.

6. Exhale and look down at the palm below your waist.

7. Inhale and look up at your extended palm above your head.

8. Exhale and very slowly, keeping your knees bent to protect your lower back, start to roll down reaching towards the ground, vertebrae by vertebrae.

9. Roll down as far as you can comfortably reach towards your toes. If you need to place your elbows on your bent knees to support your lower back, do so.

10. Hang in this position for two or three breaths, deeply breathing in through your nose and out through your mouth.

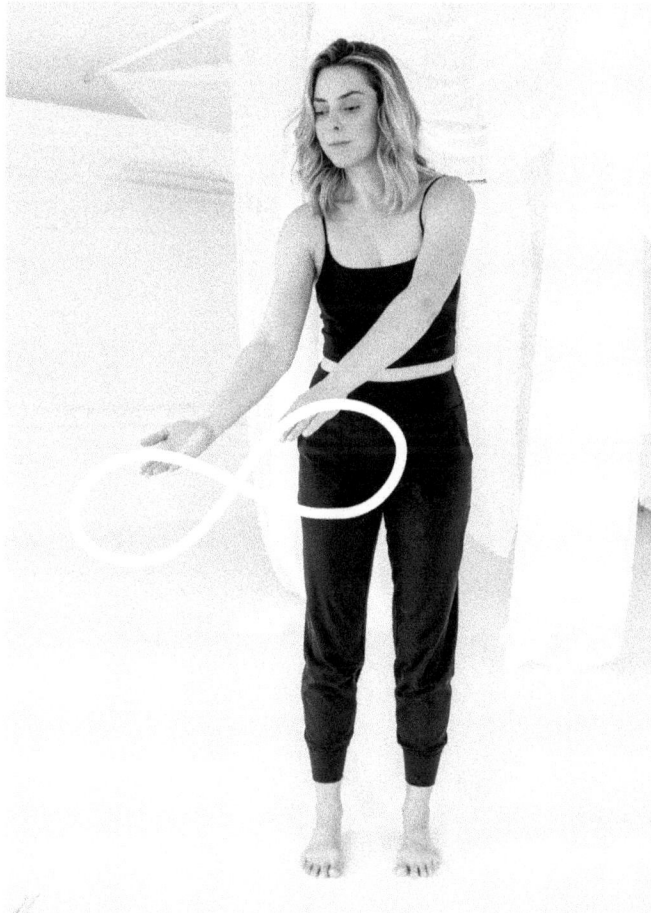

11. On your next inhale, very slowly, vertebrae by vertebrae, roll up to a standing position making big figure-eight patterns with your arms all around your body as you come up.
12. Make large and small figure-eight patterns in every direction as you come to a full standing position.
13. Extend your arms above your head as you finish making figure eights. End by expanding your arms out to the sides.
14. Do the exercise a second time.

Fatigue

Fatigue is a constant companion when undergoing cancer treatment. I found the best approach was to accept it and not resist what was inevitable. Remembering our puppy example, when animals get sick, they instinctively know they need to rest in order to heal. Certainly, post chemo, your body needs to rest, but after a while, you can get stuck in Zombieland and not know how to extricate yourself. The following are some things you can do to jump-start your energies so you can function better.

Homolateral Correction

This correction is explained in depth on Page 105.

The Four Thumps

When: Anytime you need more energy.

Why: When we are stressed, the meridians in our body start to run backwards. Having the meridians run backwards is nature's way of slowing us down, but many times, we can't or don't slow down and rest. We don't understand what is happening energetically —we just feel tired.

Since kidney meridian is the first of the 14 meridians, tapping its endpoint will jump-start all 14 meridians, getting them to flow in the right direction. Tapping on the thymus gland can help the body produce T cells and strengthen the immune system. Tapping the spleen meridian endpoints under the arms can help strengthen the immune system and enhance metabolism.

Finally, tapping on Stomach 1 will help the body stay grounded so it's less likely to go into fight, flight, or freeze mode.

How:

It's easiest to start at the top of the body and move down from there.

Stomach

1. Find the highest point on your cheekbones in line with your eyes and tap here lightly. (Since it is on your face, do not thump here, just tap.)
2. Inhale through your nose and exhale through your mouth as you tap.
3. Do this for about 30 seconds.

Kidney

1. Find your sternoclavicular notch. This is where the sternum meets your clavicle near your neck.
2. Drop down one inch to the space in between your first and second ribs. This is the last point on kidney meridian—Kidney 27.
3. Thump this point with all of your fingers with some force.
4. Inhale through your nose and exhale through your mouth.
5. Do this for about 30 seconds.

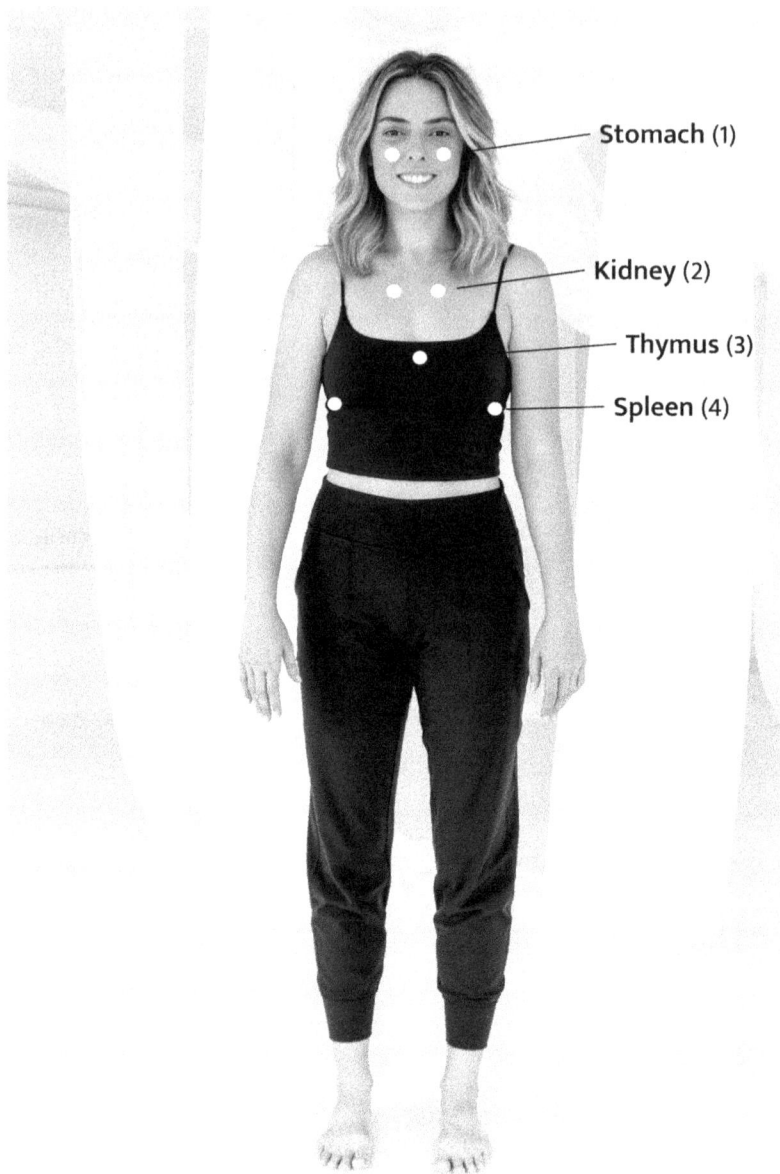

Stomach (1)

Kidney (2)

Thymus (3)

Spleen (4)

Thymus

1. Drop down to the center of your chest, in between your nipples.
2. Inhale through your nose and exhale through your mouth
3. Thump here for another 30 seconds.

Spleen

1. Extend your arms up out to your sides.
2. Find the points located on both sides of your ribcage about four inches down from your armpit.
3. Thump here for another 30 seconds.

Chemo Brain/Memory Issues

There are many supplements that could be beneficial to counteract this issue so having a consultation with a naturopath, nutritionist, or functional medicine doctor can be extremely helpful.

Two of the best EEM exercises to counteract brain fog are *Cook's Cross* (See Page 111) and *Holding the Main Neurovasculars* (See Page 97). Do these at least twice daily to help repattern the brain's right and left hemispheres' energies and to allow the blood, oxygen, and chi to remain in the brain.

Anxiety/Depression

Ricocheting between anxiety, anger, and depression is commonplace while on the cancer roller-coaster ride. Our bodies are no longer our own. Normalcy is a fleeting memory of time past. Not knowing what lies around the corner or how our body will respond triggers feelings of powerlessness, overwhelm, and frustration. Every new test or procedure post-treatment triggers the specter of a returning or new cancer. A substantial number of cancer patients and survivors are on antianxiety or antidepression medications, but these bring their own side effects such as weight gain, memory loss, and dependency. How can we deal with these emotions without medication? Activities like yoga, meditation, qigong, or massage done consistently can help, but so can EEM—and it's free! My number one technique to help counteract depression was the *homolateral correction* described in *Mounting a Defense* (See Page 105). Here are some others that can help.

Releasing the Venom

When: Whenever you feel angry, frustrated or overwhelmed.

Why: Getting unwelcome news, spending hours at the hospital, or struggling with side effects—these are just a few of the things that can make us feel frustrated and overwhelmed. These emotions get trapped not just in the mind, but in the tissue, muscles, and cells of the body. Not releasing this stuck energy can create more problems like muscle pain and headaches. Over time, chronically stuck emotions can produce illness.

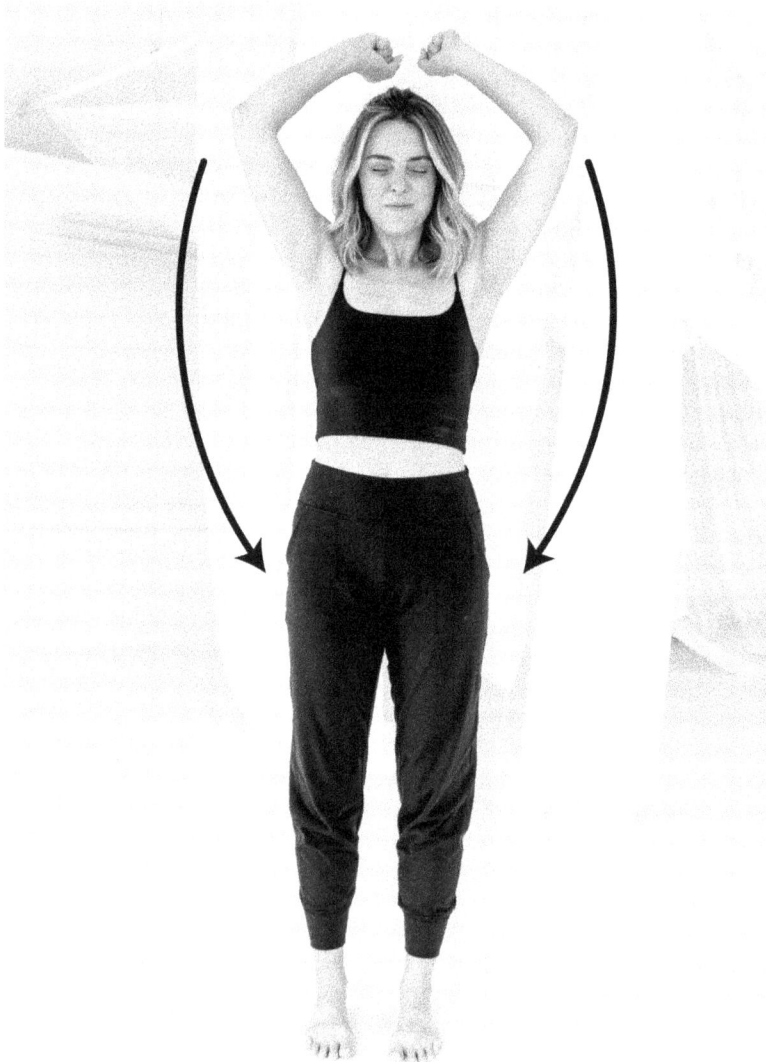

In TCM, every emotion is associated with an element, and the emotion of anger and frustration is governed by the wood element. There is also a sound associated with each element, and the sound for wood is the SHHHH sound. This exercise allows you to release that pent-up energy and move it out of the body.

How: Typically, this exercise is done standing up, but it can be done sitting down:

1. Extend your arms out in front of you. Open your palms and imagine you are placing whatever is annoying, frustrating, or upsetting into your palms.
2. Close your palms, inhale, and raise your hands up over your head.
3. With some force, release your hands down in front of you towards the floor while making a loud SHHH sound as you exhale.
4. Imagine you are releasing the pent-up emotion from your body. I like to imagine the released energy is going back into the earth to be recycled.
5. Do this exercise two more times, making a strong SHHH sound as you release the emotion through your hands.
6. On the fourth time, do the same motion, but this time move very slowly and make a soft SHHH sound imagining that what remains of the blocked emotion is fully and finally leaving your body.

Tapping the Gamut Point

When: Whenever you feel fear, panic, or anxiety.

Why: When we feel panic or anxiety, the brain's limbic system shifts into high gear. Tapping mimics the heartbeat, so the body will respond to tapping. When you tap on this triple warmer point while placing your hand over your heart, you shift the focus of the limbic system away from the brain and into the heart chakra, where more peaceful thoughts can take root. This can allow the body to calm down.

How:

1. Find the space on top of your hand in between your middle and ring finger. This is Triple Warmer 4.
2. Place your hand over your heart.
3. Tap on the Triple Warmer 4 point while breathing in through your nose and out through your mouth.

4. Do this for a count of ten.

5. Stop for a count of ten.

6. Then resume for a count of ten.

7. Do a few more rounds like this.

8. Then switch hands and repeat several rounds with the other hand.

9. You can do this for as long as it's necessary in order for you to calm down.

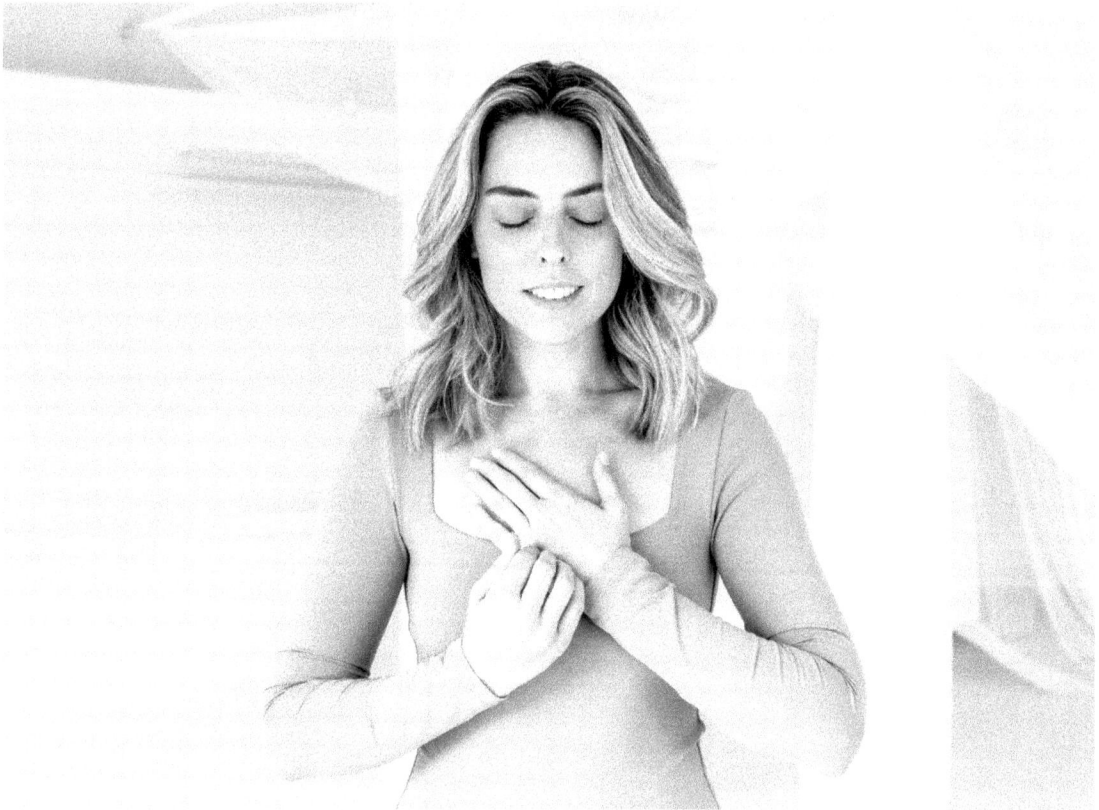

Shoulder Pull

When: Whenever you need to be grounded or come back to yourself.

Why: Our energies go homolateral when we get stressed and can get stuck there, so anything that encourages a crossover pattern (See *Homolateral Correction* on Page 105) will start to correct this pattern. Massaging the trapezoid muscles helps to calm triple warmer because the meridian runs through the muscle.

How:

1. Start by bringing your right hand to your left shoulder. Press in and massage your trapezoid muscle for about 30 seconds.
2. Now push in and drag your hand across your body to your right hip.
3. Do this another two times, moving from your left shoulder to your right hip.
4. Switch to the opposite side, massaging your right trapezius muscle with your left hand.
5. Drag your hand from the right shoulder to your left side hip.
6. Do this two more times.

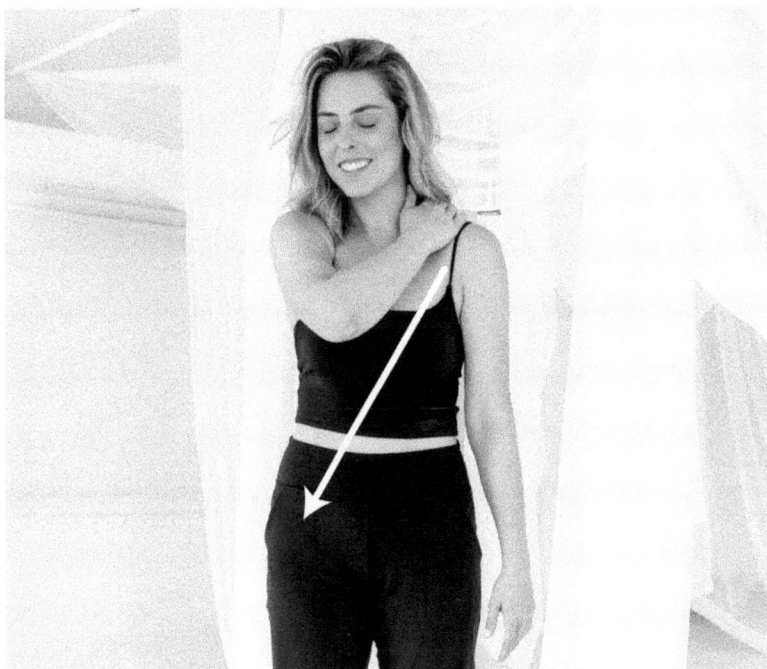

Belt Flow

When: Whenever you need to feel more grounded and embodied.

Why: As another consequence of the fight, flight, or freeze response, our body can become ungrounded. You might have heard someone say about a stressful event, "I left my body." That sensation is a consequence of trauma and can manifest as feeling agitated, spacey, confused, scared, or depressed. Doing this exercise is one of the best ways to ground yourself. It is also a radiant circuit so doing the exercise helps to reconnect the top and bottom, the front and back, and the sides of the body.

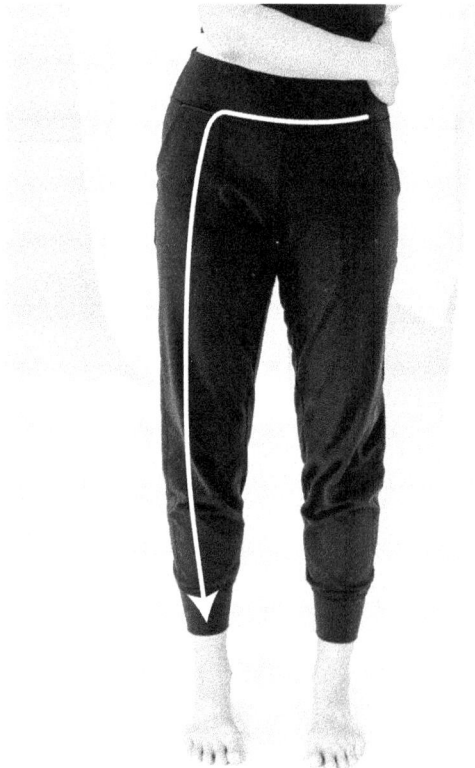

How: This should be done standing up, but it can be done sitting down if needed.

1. Take both of your hands and reach as far as you can around the left side of your waist towards the back of your body.

2. Drag your hands from your left side, across the front of your body over to your right hip.

3. Repeat this pulling and dragging motion three more times ending with both of your hands on top of your right hip bone.

4. Using your full, flat hands, smooth them down the side of your right leg, taking the energy off your right foot.

5. Do this routine one more time. Pull and drag three times, drawing the energy down the right leg and off the foot.

6. Now switch to the other side.

7. Reach both hands as far as you can to the right side of your back and waist, and drag them over to your left hip bone. Do this three times.

8. Draw your full, flat hands down the left leg, and take the energy off your left foot.

9. Do the exercise one more time on the left side.

Chapter 13

Preparation and Surgery

I received the news from my cardiologist that I had a significant arrythmia and needed a pace-maker. That was a big thing to wrap my head around. Two seconds later I felt immense relief that someone had finally found out why I was not able to walk normally for 20 paces without feeling a flush of muscle fatigue from my neck to my ankles.

Even though I was seen by a top cardiologist, and the procedure would be at a hospital known for excellent cardiac care, I still had some anxiety about having the implant. Fortunately, a friend recommended seeing an energy medicine practitioner who lived in my area.

I saw Dianne before the procedure, and she did an extensive workover, which left me far more comfortable and more confident about the procedure. The best part about the treatment is that she gave me energy 'exercises' to do at home to prepare my body to receive the pacer and also to heal more quickly after the procedure. I faithfully did the daily exercises.

I was pleasantly surprised one week after the procedure, when I had the incision check, and was told, "Your healing is perfect." I wasn't expecting such a good result from my 73-year-old body.

At that same checkup I was given the unpleasant news that shortly after the implant, I had had a lengthy Atrial Fibrillation (Afib) event (when the heartbeats are rapid and erratic, increasing the possi-bility of forming blood clots that could cause stroke). The cardiology department knows the details of my heartbeats because my pacer regularly downloads my cardiac record to a device that sits in my bedroom. That information is then transferred to the cardiology department. I was advised to begin an anti-co-agulant drug – what they call blood thinners - to prevent stroke. I decided to wait another month to see if the incidence of Afib recurred. In the meantime, I received another treatment from Dianne, and she gave me daily energy healing exercises to smooth the heartbeats and to strengthen the heart energy circuit.

So far, 9 months later, there have been no further incidents of Afib.

I feel so fortunate that I found out about energy medicine and had this support through my cardiac procedure and the healing process.

Carol M.

When I looked back at my cancer journey, surgery was the most manageable of the three treatments. It only lasted a day, and I had medication to numb the pain so I could slowly heal my wounds. It certainly wasn't a walk in the park, but compared to chemo and radiation, it was the least traumatic and debilitating even though it was an amputation of sorts. Because I had a PT who specialized in lymphedema, I never developed it. Otherwise perhaps my story would be quite different. More than a year later, I had full range of motion with my arm, little pain, and minimal numbness. I diligently did yoga, stretching, or qigong to help the muscles and tissues maintain their suppleness and flexibility.

The Eden Method has a series of energy interventions it recommends prior to and after surgery. Some of these have been mentioned in Chapters 11 and 12, but they are equally as important for surgery. Ideally, a caregiver would help if possible.

Preparation for Surgery

Homolateral Energies

Your body will go homolateral due to the surgery. If you can, do the homolateral correction at least twice a day. (See Page 105) If you can't stand, do it sitting or lying down. Or if you don't have the energy to muster that, draw figure eights around your eyes slowly with your pointer finger for at least a minute or two.

Tibetan Rings

Why: Tibetan rings are named for a healing technique Tibetans have used for centuries. An energy configuration that sits just off the body, tibetan rings follow the body's anatomy to strengthen and reinforce it. The tibetan rings are shaped like the number eight. If one is broken, it can impact the integrity of that body part. For example, prior to my surgery, my daughter tested the tibetan ring over my right breast and it was consistently broken.

The main ones are located bilaterally from the shoulder to the hip, from the hip to the feet on the front and back of the body, and on each surface of the head, hands, feet and ankles.

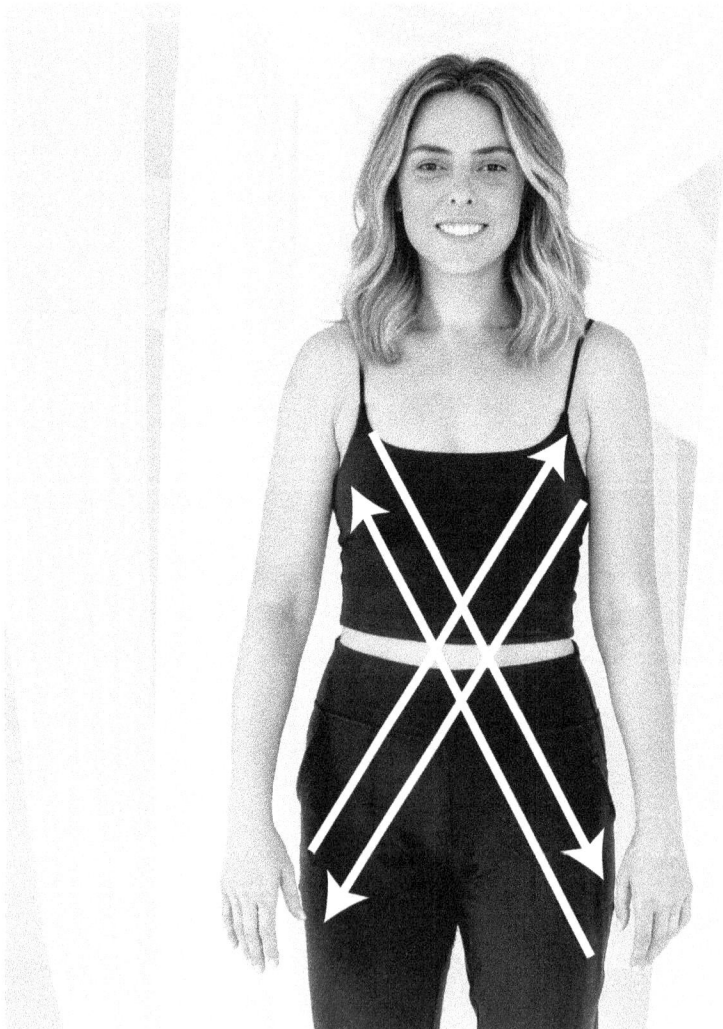

How:

1. Starting at the shoulder, swipe down to the opposite hip. Test.
2. Now swipe up from the hip to the shoulder. Test.
3. Do the same thing on the opposite shoulder.
4. Do this test on any body part or organ that may be compromised.
5. If either one of those directions tests weak, it means the energy is not flowing properly in that direction.

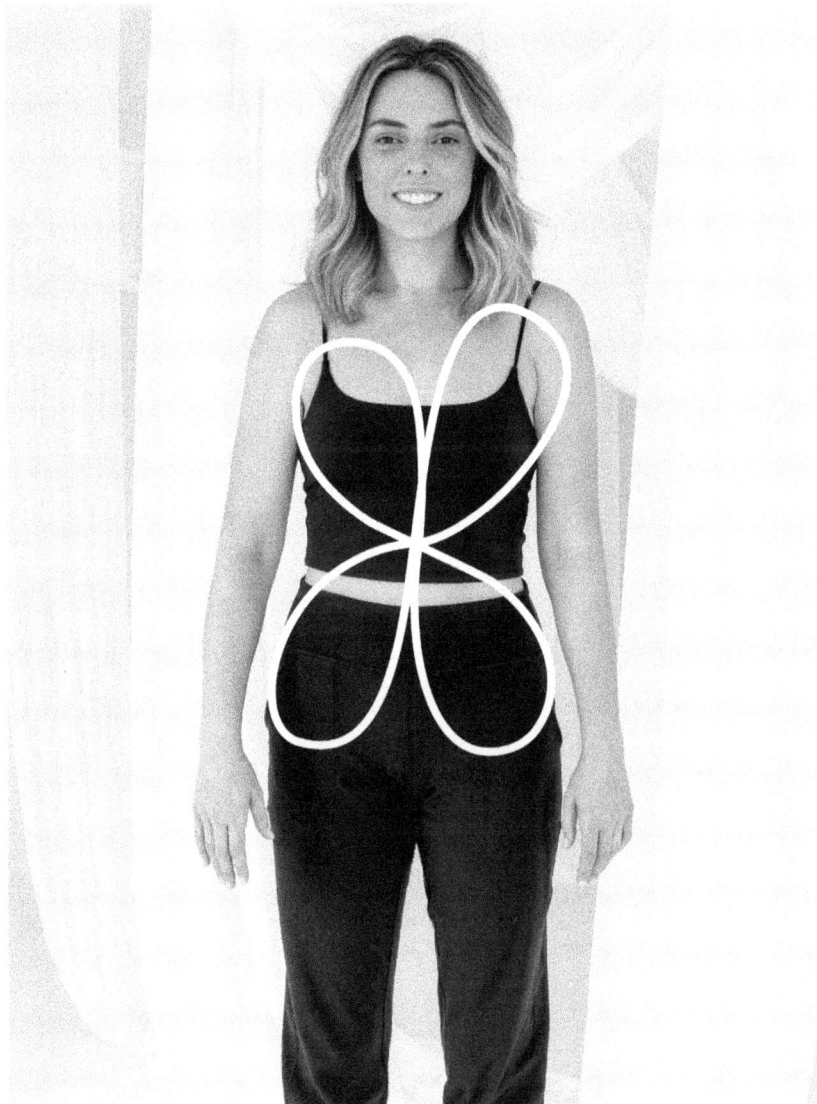

4. To mend the break, start by drawing figure eight patterns in the direction that tested strong and then move into the direction that tested weak. It's sort of like catching a wave: starting with the strong direction will facilitate the energy to move into the weak area.

5. Do at least seven or eight passes to correct the break.

6. Do twice daily until the pattern can hold.

If you don't know how to energy test or don't feel confident doing so, you can simply make these large and small patterns a few inches of the body, paying particular attention to your area of weakness. This will both reinforce the body's anatomy and the biofield itself. I had a cancer client whose spouse would spend a half-hour every day making figure eights around him to fortify his energies throughout his cancer treatment. She continues to do this even to this day!

Clearing and Strengthening Chakras

This technique is explained in detail on Page 132. Since surgery directly impacts the chakras, have someone do this prior to and after surgery.

Holding Meridian Neurovascular Points

When: Before and after surgery daily.

Why: Every meridian in the body has positive and negative emotions associated with it. These emotions can be accessed by working with neurovascular points on the head that correspond to these emotional centers. Holding these points lightly can balance negative emotions and help keep the body calm before and after surgery.

I attended an EEM conference many years ago where a young came to the podium and said he had been diagnosed with a malignant brain tumor. He decided to hold all of his neurovascular points every day for two months. The next time he went in for a scan, his tumor was gone! He was convinced it was holding his neurovasculars that made the difference.

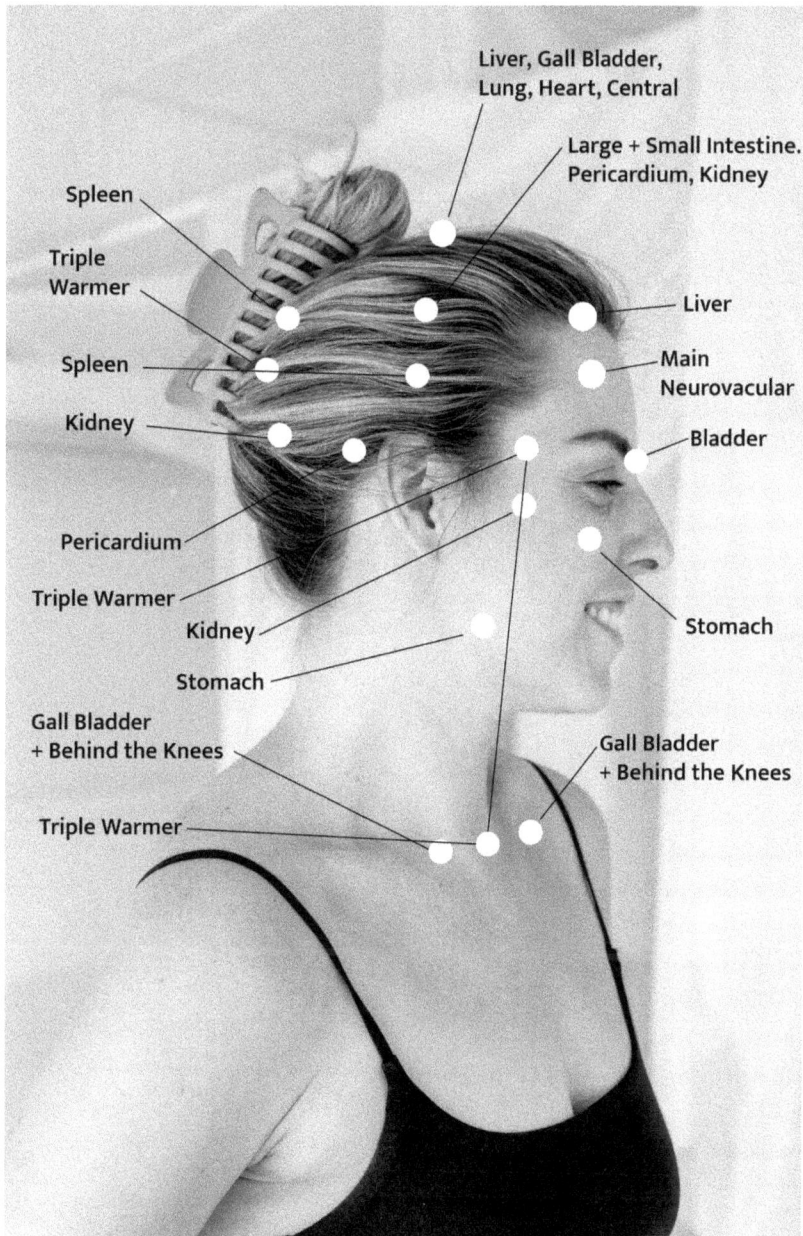

You can hold the neurovascular points that align for your particular cancer. Because an imbalance between your spleen and triple warmer energies is always at the heart of an immune dysfunction, you should hold those neurovascular points as well.

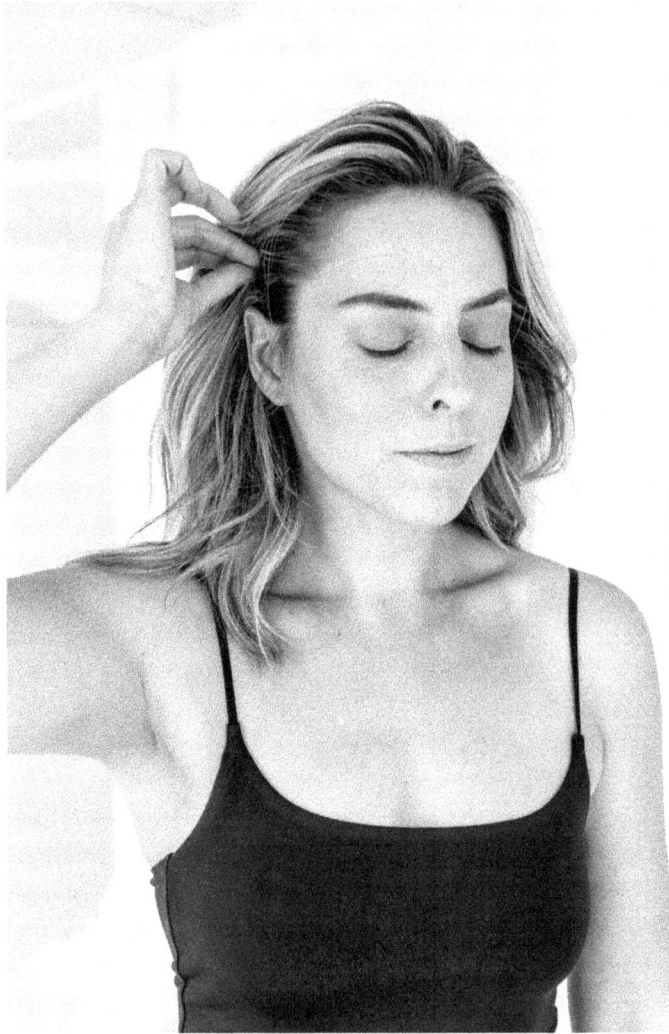

How:

1. The easiest way to hold these points is to take your thumb, pointer, and middle finger and place them lightly on the point. Of course, the ideal would be to have someone do this for you.

2. Hold each point for at least three minutes once or twice a day. You cannot "overdo" holding these points. They are like the radiant circuits; the longer you hold them, the deeper they will go. If they are bilateral, hold on each side.

3. Here are some common cancers and their corresponding neurovascular points:

Bone – kidney and bladder

Brain – all of the neurovasculars held one at a time or those that are

closest to the tumor's location

Breast – stomach, spleen, and pericardium

Colon – large and small intestine and lung

Endometrial – liver and pericardium

Leukemia – heart, spleen, and pericardium

Lung - lung and large intestine

Lymphoma – spleen and triple warmer

Melanoma – lung and large intestine

Ovarian – pericardium

Pancreatic – spleen

Prostate – kidney, bladder, and pericardium

Source Points

When: Perform before and after surgery.

Why: Source points are acupuncture points that can help revitalize the body after an illness or before and after surgery. They are located where the primordial energy in the meridians pool and therefore contain concentrated amounts of chi. They are called source points because they directly "source" energy to the organ for which they are named. Massaging, tapping, spinning a crystal, or figure eighting these points are ways to send energy directly to the stressed, diseased or otherwise compromised organ. Since illness is reflected in reversed polarity somewhere along the meridian line, you will start with rebalancing the source point's polarity.

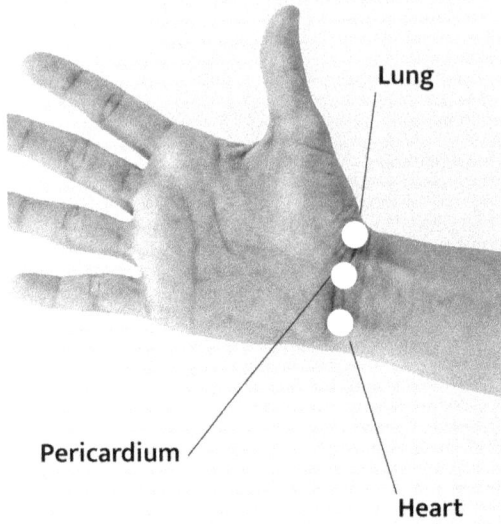

Lung

Pericardium

Heart

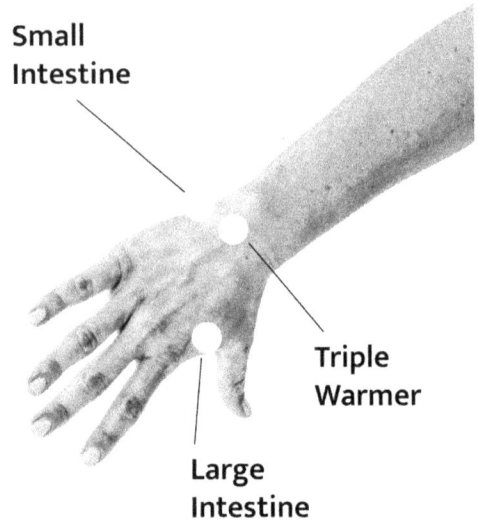

Small Intestine

Triple Warmer

Large Intestine

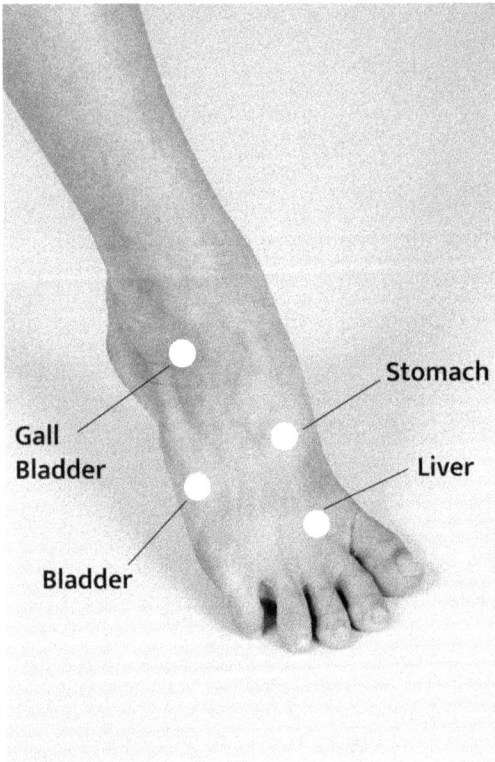

Gall Bladder

Stomach

Liver

Bladder

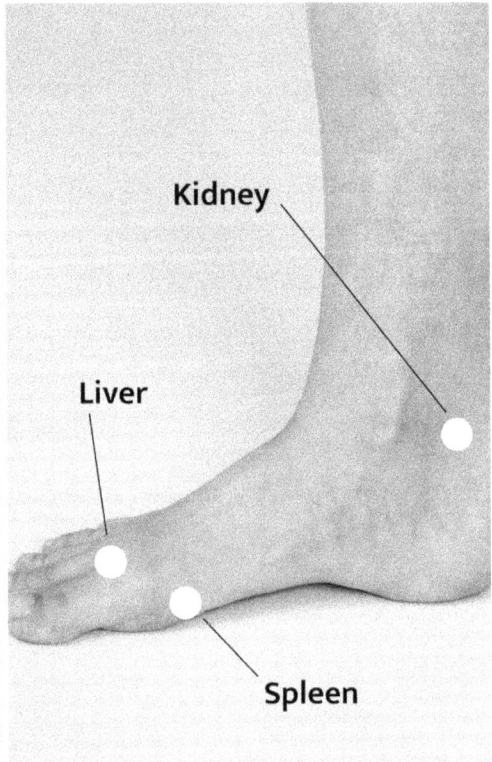

Kidney

Liver

Spleen

How:

To balance the point's polarity, start by either spinning a crystal or flipping your fingers back and forth on each point for a couple of seconds.

1. You can work with just the source point corresponding to your cancer, or you can do a series of holds on each point to help revitalize the body.
2. Each meridian in the body has a time period associated with it.
3. Start with the point that corresponds to the present time of day. Each time period is marked on the chart below. For example, if it's 11 a.m., you will start with heart source point.

Time	Meridian
11 AM – 1 PM	Heart
1 PM – 3 PM	Small Intestine
3 PM – 5 PM	Bladder
5 PM – 7 PM	Kidney
7 PM – 9 PM	Pericardium
9 PM – 11 PM`	Triple Warmer
11 PM – 1 AM	Gall Bladder
1 AM – 3 AM	Liver
3 AM – 5 AM	Lung
5 AM – 7 AM	Large Intestine
7 AM - 9 AM	Stomach
9 AM – 11 AM	Spleen

4. Massage, tap or figure eight this point for at least 30 seconds to a minute.
5. Do both the right and left sides of the body before moving to the next point.
6. Move around the clock and massage, tap, or figure eight each of these points until you have completed the 24-hour clock.

Post-Surgery: Healing the Body

Continue to have someone do *chakra clearing* (See Page 132), *neurovascular* (See page 166), or *source point* (See Page 169) work at least weekly and preferably more often. When I worked with my cancer clients, their caregivers were working on them daily during their treatments, sometimes for up to an hour. Continue to correct for homolateral energies and strengthen your biofield by making large and small figure eights around your body daily.

Shock Points

Holding or having someone hold your shock points will allow your body to process and release the surgical trauma.

When: It can and should be done throughout your cancer treatments.

Why: Shock enters the body through three points located on the soles of the feet. Just as an electrical shock can wreak havoc on an appliance, energetic shock from a surgery, car accident or medical procedure can wreak havoc on the body. The shock reverberates throughout the nervous system and triple warmer attempts to process it but is not always successful. You might know someone who was in a car accident and never felt the same afterwards. Or someone who had surgery and was told it was successful, but they never fully recovered. Releasing the residual shock from the body can help the nervous system come back into balance.

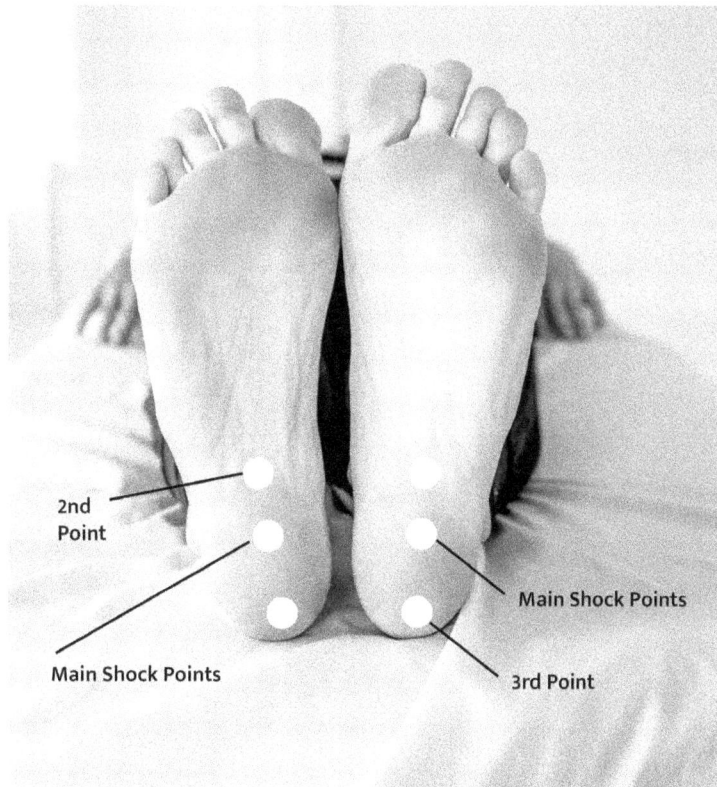

How: Ideally, someone would hold these points for you because there needs to be a fair amount of pressure exerted. There are three shock points located vertically on the heel. The main point is in the center of the heel, the second is distal to the main point (at the base of the heel), and the third one is at the top of the heel.

Protocol: Written from the practitioner's perspective

1. The recipient will need to be sitting upright with their feet extended or lying down with their feet easily accessible.
2. *Open the gaits* of your hands. (See Page 105)
3. *Open the gaits* of the recipient's feet, paying particular attention to the soles of the feet, including the heels.
4. *Spoon the feet* (See Page 110) to balance the polarity.
5. Find the middle of the recipient's heels and imagine there is a bullseye located there.
6. With pressure, push into that center point. (6-8 on a scale of 0–10)

7. Hold for a couple of minutes.

8. You can do both points at the same time, or you can work on one point at a time. Always check in with your recipient to make sure the pressure is OK.

9. Move to the second set of points at the base of the heels and push in hard here.

10. Hold for another couple of minutes.

11. Move to the third set of points and press hard.

12. Hold for another couple of minutes.

Jin Shin Jitsu

Jin Shin Jitsu is an ancient Japanese healing technique that was rediscovered in the 20th century by Jiro Murai and brought to the West by Mary Bermeister.

When: It can be performed by anyone at any time. It's something to do when you have very little stamina or feel ill. It's also a terrific way to fall asleep.

Why: Each finger is the beginning or end point of a meridian, so each finger is a gateway to the energy and function of those meridians. Holding the fingers individually accesses those meridians and the physical, mental, and emotional properties associated with them. There are studies showing that cancer patients who used this practice during their treatment had less overall pain and anxiety.[16]

How: I have seen this technique taught in different ways. You can either work with one hand at a time, or you can go back and forth between hands as you move through the individual fingers. This explanation uses the latter method and for clarification will start with the left hand. Slowing down your breathing brings the nervous system into alignment with the energetic shifts that the holds are creating, so try to do five-second inhale/six-second-exhale breathing if possible.

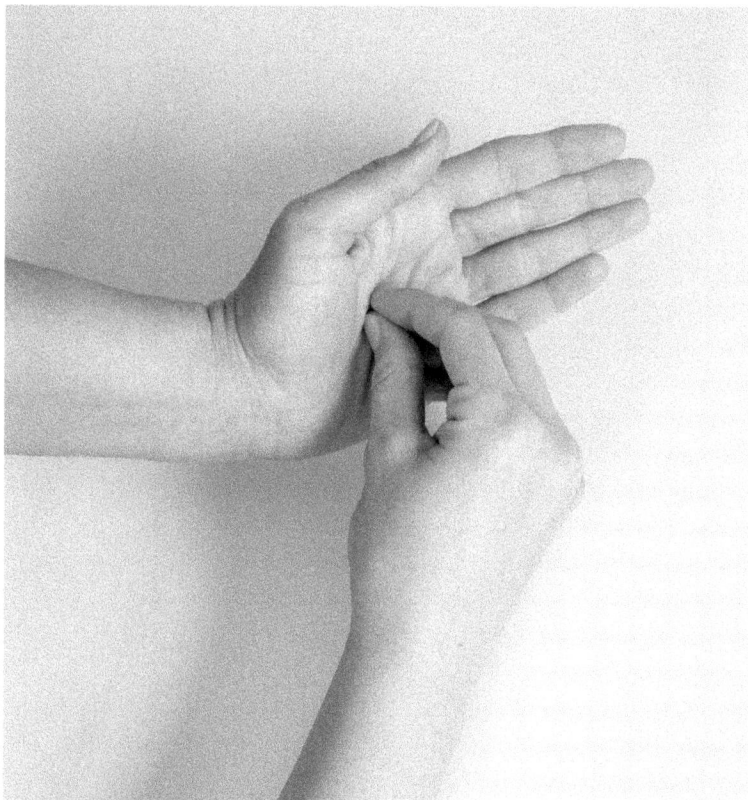

1. Place the thumb, pointer, and middle fingers of your right hand into the center of the left palm.

2. Hold for one to three minutes.

3. Switch hands and take the thumb, pointer, and middle finger of your left hand and place them inside the right palm.

4. Hold for one to three minutes.

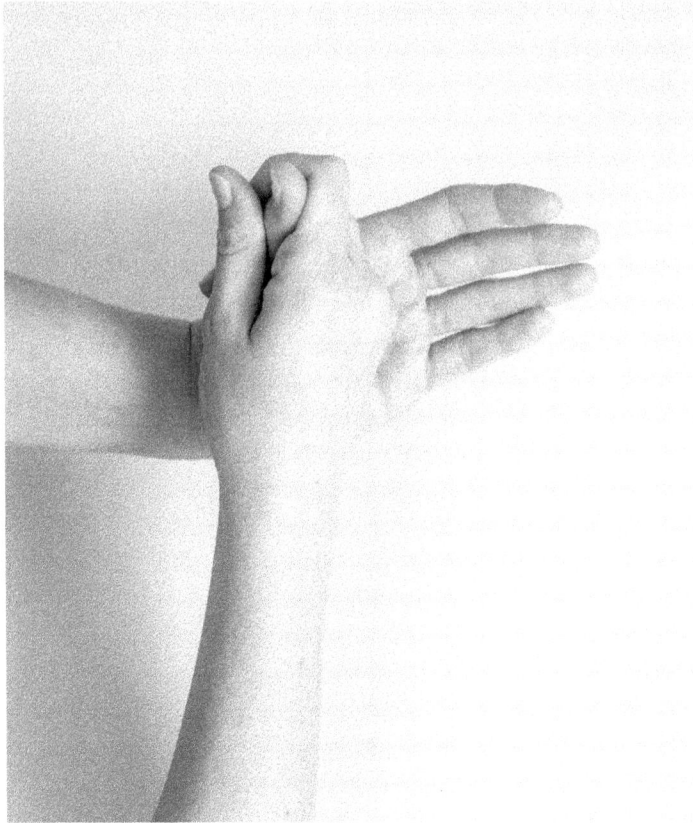

5. Take the fingers of your left hand and hold your right thumb.

6. Hold one to three minutes.

7. Switch sides and hold your left thumb with the fingers of your right hand.

8. Hold one to three minutes.

9. Hold your left pointer finger with the fingers of your right hand.

10. Hold one to three minutes.

11. Switch sides and hold the right pointer finger with the fingers of your left hand.

12. Hold one to three minutes.

13. Hold your right middle finger with the fingers of your left hand.

14. Hold one to three minutes.

15. Switch sides and hold your left middle finger with your right hand.

16. Hold one to three minutes.

17. Hold your left ring finger with the fingers of your right hand.

18. Hold one to three minutes.

19. Switch sides and hold your right ring finger with the fingers of your left hand.

20. Hold one to three minutes.

21. Hold your right little finger with the fingers of your left hand.

22. Hold one to three minutes.

23. Switch sides and hold your left little finger with the fingers of your right hand.

24. Hold one to three minutes.

Play with this format to see which feels better for you: Holding all the fingers of one hand first, or switching back and forth and holding each finger on each side. Don't feel compelled to move to the next finger. When I did this technique, I never considered the time. I just tuned into my body to see what felt the best. Sometimes one finger needed to be held longer than another, perhaps up to five minutes. If you hold the fingers a longer time, you may begin to feel a pulsing or tingling sensation as the blood, oxygen, and energy move through your fingers and meridian lines.

Scars

All of the medical professionals who have examined my scar mentioned how wonderful it looks. Not that I'm proud of it, but unlike many I have seen online, mine is not raised, discolored or contractured. It is narrow and, a year post-surgery, only slightly numb. I attribute this to not just my amazing, super young surgeon, but also to my skin care and energy medicine. Even today, I put a natural oil on the scar daily to keep it from tightening up and helping to keep the skin supple. I also do yoga and weightlifting to keep the muscles around it strong.

Figure Eighting

When: Perform daily post-surgery until the scar fully heals.

Why: Scars create blockage in the energy field and prevent the chi from moving freely, so figure eighting the scar can help move some of the blockage through. From the first week post-surgery, I used a cut-glass crystal in front of my scar daily. Spinning a cut-glass crystal helps to break up whatever energetic congestion has formed in the biofield around the incision. Breaking up that stuck energy can help the skin heal faster and better. I continued to do this for about the first year post-surgery.

How:

1. Starting about three inches off the body, spin the crystal back and forth over the entire length of the scar.
2. Do this several times in each direction.
3. Do it a couple of times and day.
4. Do it preventatively over the course of the following year or whenever you feel pulling or tautness at the site.

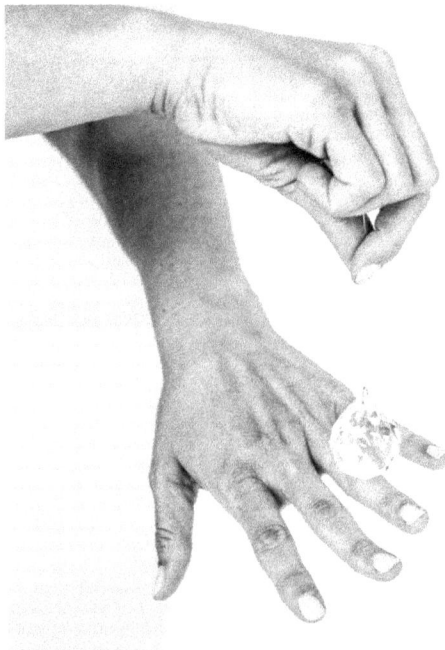

Chapter 14

Radiation

My cancer diagnosis came as a shock to me. I had been suffering from unexplained swelling that no one could figure out. Finally, a doctor thought it might be a bacterial infection and ordered a CT scan. To his surprise, he found out that I had Stage 4 cancer with a bleak outlook. A cancer team confirmed that my only chance was drastic surgery that would leave me disabled.

As I contemplated my next steps with my wife, I met Dianne, an Eden Energy Medicine (EEM) Practitioner. She conducted a thorough interview and energy testing on me and determined that certain pathways in my immune system were not functioning properly. That was followed by immediate in-office energy treatment and concluded with a list of exercises, meditations and home treatments that my wife could perform to aid in my recovery.

While receiving a cancer diagnosis can leave one feeling helpless and powerless, Dianne's extensive knowledge and application of EEM provided me with the tools and structure to cope with the illness and the overwhelming psychological pressure that comes with it. I followed a daily routine exercise to keep my energies unified while my wife faithfully performed home treatments every evening. Dianne also taught me self-affirming meditations to calm my mind and help me sleep, which were also useful during the long diagnostic scans and chemotherapy treatments.

EEM provided the foundation for my recovery. As I sought additional options from other doctors, they noticed my energy and vigor and seemed to provide me with a higher level of care as a result. In the end, I was able to avoid the debilitating surgery and make a full recovery despite the side effects from the chemoradiation treatment. I credit Dianne's expert diagnosis and use of EEM for providing the foundation for my recovery and giving me the tools to overcome this seemingly insurmountable challenge. I am thankful for the profound impact of energy on my health and the impact it has had

on every aspect of my life.
    Andy H.

In Chapter Five, I describe how difficult radiation was for me, even from Day One. Energy testing showed that many systems were out of balance after each session, including:

1. Energies were not crossing over.
2. Holes and tears were in the biofield.
3. Chakras were weak and imbalanced.
4. Neurological energies were scrambled.
5. Shock points were weak.
6. Triple warmer was reactive.
7. Radiant circuit energies were dormant.
8. Tibetan Rings were off.

This was happening every day. At first, I didn't understand exactly what was happening energetically; I just felt depressed, angry, and vulnerable. I was shocked when I learned how quickly the radiation was affecting my energies, even someone like me who knew, understood, and practiced energy medicine. Fortunately, I had energy medicine tools that could help me reverse and manage these symptoms.

The corrections for each of these issues has already been presented in earlier chapters:

1. Homolateral Correction – Page 128
2. Figure Eights – Page 147
3. Clearing and Strengthening Chakras – Page 132
4. Cooks Cross Correction - Page 111
5. Shock Point Correction – Page 172
6. Mellow Mudra and Main Neurovascular Hold – Page 98
7. Holding Radiant Circuit Points – Page 115
8. Tibetan Rings – Page 164

Once I realized my energies needed to be attended to quickly and regularly to protect myself, I was diligent about doing Numbers 1, 2, 4, and 6 prior to and after treatment. In fact, I would go to a quiet place just before entering the radiation room and do the holds; then I would go back to the quiet place afterwards and hold them again before driving home. That night, I would have Kim clear and strengthen my chakras, hold my shock points, and reactivate my radiant circuits. I also found that holding my neurovasculars was helpful. In particular, I held triple warmer, spleen, and stomach points. (See Page 166.)

Despite our best efforts, however, over time even these exercises no longer worked. It was at this point that I started to feel my life force being pulled from my body and not knowing if I had the strength to carry on. This was also when my immune system started to break down. Kim and I struggled to know what to do. How could we use EEM to combat the energy that was penetrating my field and body?

Then it dawned on us: We could use color to combat color! Every day, I had two color beams infiltrating my body during radiation: One was red, and one was green. These beams would turn off and on, alternating over the course of the 15-minute session.

Kim energy tested to find out what colors could counteract the radiation that was entering my body. Sometimes it needed blue; sometimes it was another color, like lavender. We used scarves of an assortment of colors and placed them on and around my body every day after my treatment. We also used specialized color flashlights. They had filters that projected the colors onto my biofield and into my chakras. This was the remarkable way my body was able to balance the daily energetic onslaught of radiation treatment. Fortunately, I didn't have to continue much longer, but the use of color was a powerful antidote to what my energy systems had absorbed from the radiation.

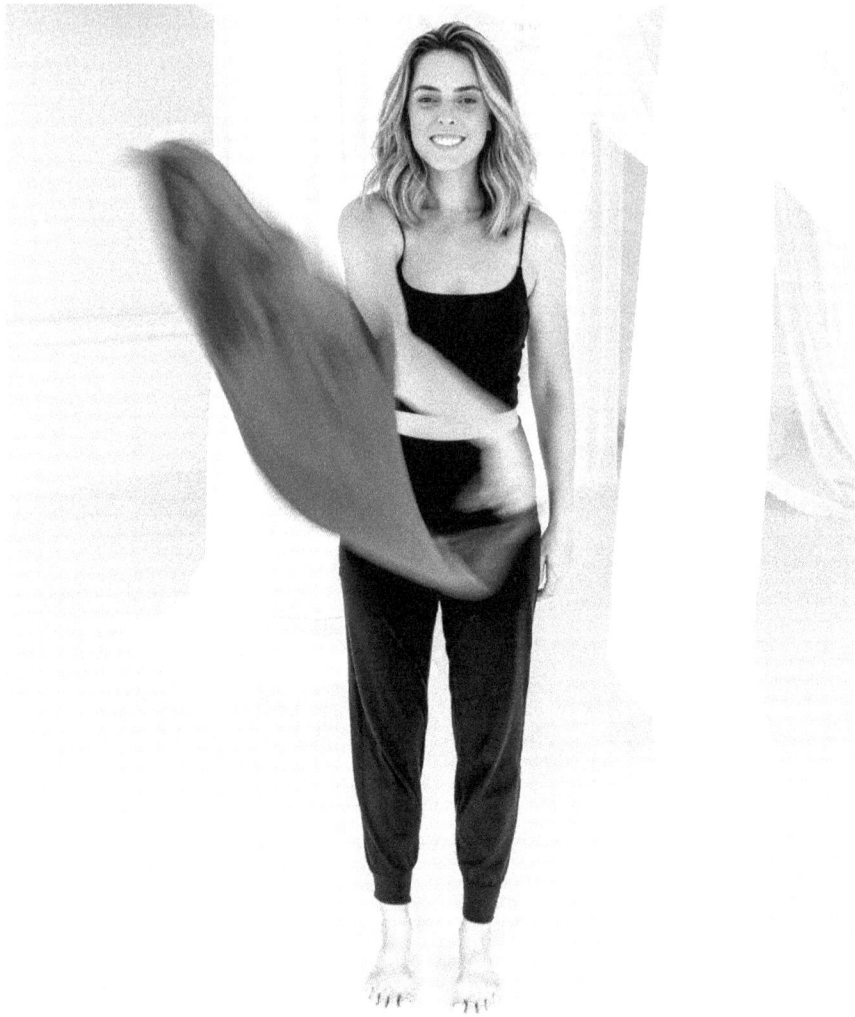

Kim's Insights on Radiation

Nothing was harder to get out of my mom's energy systems than the daily onslaught of radiation. We could barely get her field back intact before the next day, and the cumulative effect of her radiation made it harder and harder as we went. My hands didn't feel like they were enough. I would clear and clear to no avail. I was inspired to take some colorful silk scarves and use them to clear the field. It seemed to be the thing that moved the needle. With one silk scarf in each hand, I would make circles outward from her body almost as if a dance. The energy shifted so much easier. It was palpable.

A couple weeks into her radiation phase, her skin got bad, really bad. By then I forgot about the silk and was pretty stressed and disconnected from my source. My weakness made me vulnerable. I would feel it coming over me starting in my hands, then up my arms, and finally as a clenching in my head—almost as if there were a vice gripping the top of my head. I couldn't shake it and had the craziest dreams that night.

A second session, and same thing. My mom had to do an energy session on me! It occurred to us both to use her colored flashlights. The effect was immediate. It cut through the artificial buzzing, thick, gooey energy immediately. After my mom cleared my energies, we used the colored flashlights on her from then on.

Chapter 15

Recovery

When I was admitted to the ICU with a diagnosis of both liver and kidney failure, I didn't know much about energy medicine, but it didn't take long for me to recognize its benefits.

My liver failure meant that my body could not filter out toxins or process vitamins so almost everything tested through blood work was dangerously out of normal range. I was jaundiced and my energy levels were near zero. My liver was leaking all fluids that I ingested into my abdomen which meant that no fluids were reaching my kidneys to be filtered or expelled. I had to have a weekly procedure called a paracentesis, which involved using a needle to extract all of the excess fluid from my abdomen. I was put on a very strict diet and put on dialysis several days per week. Needless to say, I was very ill. In fact, I was given less than a 50% chance to live beyond three months. I was told that I would need a liver transplant if I survived.

I was not getting better, so I decided to contact Dianne. After my first visit, I was surprised at how much she could tell me about my personality and how I deal with situations just by energy testing. After my second visit, I felt noticeably stronger and more energized. But the third visit is when I absolutely knew that the energy work was helping. As I was on the table being worked on, I felt a physical sensation in my kidneys and ever since I have been able to urinate properly and consistently. The fluid buildup stopped and I no longer needed paracentesis. I was off dialysis in just a few weeks.

Today, my blood work is normal, my energy levels are up, I no longer have jaundice and I feel great. I no longer need a liver transplant. There is no doubt that energy medicine saved my life.

Jon B.

When I first envisioned this book, I failed to recognize that the chapters designed to assist one's journey through cancer treatment—chemotherapy, surgery, and radiation—were lacking a fourth and equally important addition: post-cancer recovery. In other words, putting the pieces back together. This is a huge issue for many people undergoing cancer treatment. It can sometimes prevent people from getting better. After registering the shock of the diagnosis, they rise to the occasion to fight the battle at hand. They do everything their doctors tell them to do. They take all the drugs, do all the procedures, and try lots of alternative treatments or supplements to rebuild their immune system, but something is not quite right. There are many ways this phenomenon can show up.

Following the Western approach to cancer treatment is dehumanizing. The continual procedures, medications, and treatments can leave one in a state of shock and depression or post-traumatic stress. One survivor stated it this way: "They cured my cancer, and I am 20 years post-treatment, but my body never recovered from the treatment." Another cancer survivor told me she has *anhedonia*—the inability to feel joy, a subset of depression. Doctors don't know why some people suffer like this after their cancer treatment. This is an area where energy medicine can be quite helpful.

Our body's sophisticated physiology is reflected in the complexities of the energies in and around it. The following could all be at play following a cancer course of treatment. Any one of these could be the cause of or a contributing factor to depression, PTSD, or anhedonia.

1. A chronic homolateral condition
2. A triple warmer imbalance
3. A radiant circuit dysfunction
4. A broken major or minor grid

If someone has been attending to their energies, keeping them crossing over and keeping triple warmer out of fight or flight, bouncing back from cancer treatment might not be too difficult. If, on the other hand, someone has been moving through their treatments without addressing the energetic fundamentals spelled out in Part ll, they might find themselves depressed, exhausted, or anxious by the end of their journey. If they continue using traditional medical approaches to their problem, they will be put on more medications, which will present their own side effects. This approach does not solve the underlying cause of the problem.

The first step is to get out of homolateral (See Page 105). It might take days, weeks, or even months, but eventually, the body will get the message not to go back into homolateral. Next is to get out of fight-or-flight response. This, too, can take a while to shift. The holds described in Part II are a good place to start, but both temporal tapping and EFT tapping can be extremely helpful to shift blocked emotions. Temporal tapping is described on Page 125. EFT could be done with a practitioner, but you can also get some relief on your own. There are many excellent resources and EFT teachers who can give a more in-depth explanation of the technique, but below is a simple first step you can use.

Emotional Freedom Technique (EFT)

When: Anytime you want to remove emotions that are negatively impacting your life.

Why: Tapping on specific acupressure points sends signals to the brain and nervous system that can interrupt or disconnect the nexus between the memory of an event, and an emotion associated with that event. The body responds to tapping because it is similar to the heartbeat. As a person taps on the issue and the emotions surrounding that issue, the relationship between the emotion and the issue, event, or memory starts to become disassociated, and eventually the connection is broken. It is a relatively fast process and can resolve problems that have not been resolved through traditional talk therapy.

How:

1. Decide what issue you want to tap on. Work on only one issue at a time. This technique focuses on the negative emotion, so choose something that is actually bothering you. For this example, I will use the issue of grief: what has been lost from the cancer experience.

2. Rate this issue on a scale of 0–10, 10 being the most triggering. If something is an actual 10, don't start with that issue. Choose something that is in the 7–8 range. (If you are aware of issues that are in the 10 range, consider working with either an EFT practitioner, life coach, or psychotherapist.)

3. Once you have identified an issue you want to work on, tune into your body and

notice where your attention is drawn while thinking about the issue. Is it your stomach? Your heart? Rate that sensation on a scale of 0-10.

4. Even though you are working with a negative memory or issue, you want to choose a positive statement to tap into the acupuncture points. You will be making this statement out loud throughout this practice. My grief, for example, I rated at a 7 on a scale of 0–10 and the statement I will be tapping is:

> *Even though I am experiencing grief as a consequence of my cancer treatment,*
> *I deeply love and accept myself.*

5. Begin by bringing the edges of your palms together—like a karate chop—(small intestine meridian) while making this statement out loud:

> *Even though I am experiencing grief as a consequence of my cancer treatment,*
> *I deeply love and accept myself.*

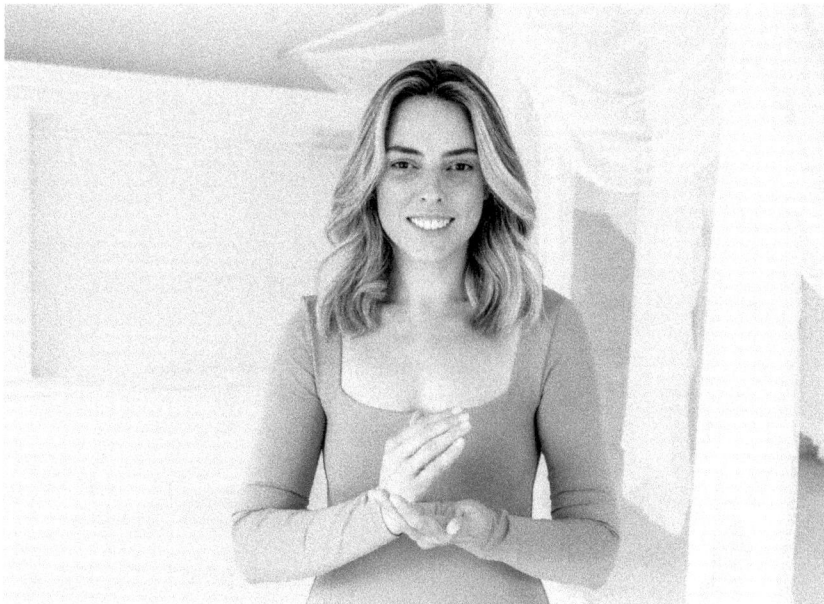

6. Continue to tap these points while making the statement at least three times. Now move to tapping the points on the head and body. You can continue to tap the statement, or you can shorten it along the lines of either of the following two statements:

It's a 7 on a scale of 0–10
Or:
This grief of mine.

7. While making these statements, tap on the following sequence of points:

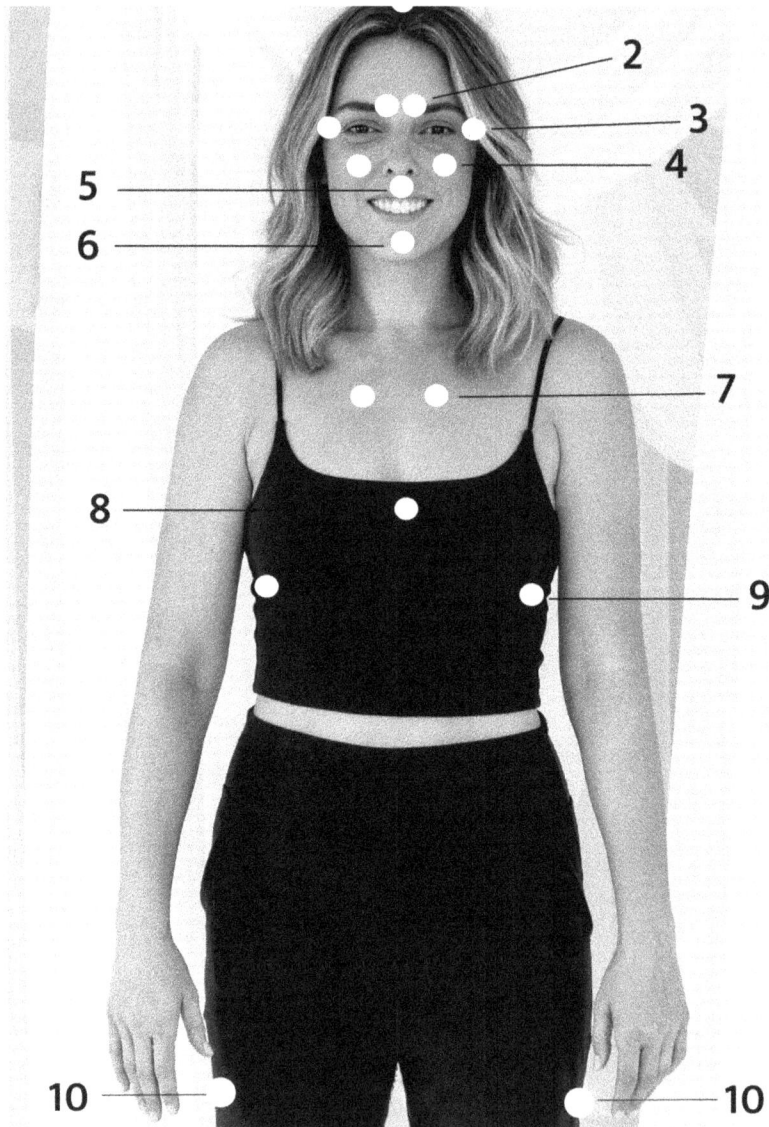

1. On top of the head (bladder and governing meridians)

2. On the inner edge of each eyebrow (bladder meridian)

3. On either side of the eyes at the temple (triple warmer and gall bladder meridians)

4. At the highest point on the cheekbone, directly in line with the pupil (stomach)

5. Upper lip - In the space between the nose and the mouth (governing meridian)

6. On the chin (central meridian)

7. Below the clavicle in the space between your collarbone and your first rib (kidney meridian)

8. At the center of the chest on the breastbone in between the nipples (central meridian and thymus gland)

9. On either side of the rib cage in line with the armpit, approximately four inches below the armpit (spleen meridian)

10. On the sides of the legs, directly where your fingers touch if you have your fingers pointing towards the leg (gall bladder meridian)

Tapping these points while making the statement constitutes one round of EFT. At the end of each round, check in with your body and see whether the initial number has moved down. For some people, it can jump down to a 2 or 3, for others it might drop down point by point, from a 7 to a 6 to a 5, and so forth, with each round.

Your goal is to get the number to a 1 or 0. If you find your number is either not dropping down at all or another memory, event or emotion shows up, stop what you are doing and focus on that emotion or memory. Rate the number for that issue and start the technique for that issue or emotion. Do one issue/emotion at a time. If you have any concerns or questions, consult with an EFT professional. There are more advanced techniques that can help shift resistant or deeper issues.

Detoxifying the Body

Once your treatments are finished, you can finally focus on getting rid of the toxins that have built up in your body for months or even years. Chemotherapy drugs are detoxified via the liver and kidneys, but the body can also use the lungs, skin, spleen, colon, and lymph system to detoxify. Using detoxification techniques can help move the residual chemo out of the body and facilitate a speedier recovery. Acupuncture can help. Exercise is good; so is anything that makes you sweat, like an infrared sauna. (Be sure to clear this with your healthcare provider first.) Skin brushing or lymphatic massage is another way to move toxins out of the body. I used bentonite clay and Epsom salt baths to help detox. Bentonite clay can also be used to detox the colon. Working with a naturopath who can prescribe herbs, supplements, or homeopathy is another option. Of course, EEM can help too.

Source Points – Massaging, tapping, or holding the source points involved in detoxifying the body is easy and sends energy directly to the organ. Ones to focus on would be liver, kidney, spleen, lung, and large intestine. (See chart on Page 170.) You want to do these daily for a couple of minutes.

Neurolymphatic Points

These points have already been discussed on Page 143. They are a direct link to activating the lymphatic system for a particular organ. Again, liver, kidney, spleen lung, and large intestine would be appropriate. Remember to use pressure on these points—between a 7 on a scale of 0–10 unless you are too weak to even withstand that amount. Start slowly if you received a lot of chemo or are still on medications. Spend a couple of minutes on these every day if possible. After a while they shouldn't hurt. That's how you know the organ has been detoxified. During the time of my treatment, my kidney point at L1 on the spine was excruciatingly painful. Now it doesn't hurt at all, but it took a year for the pain to go away.

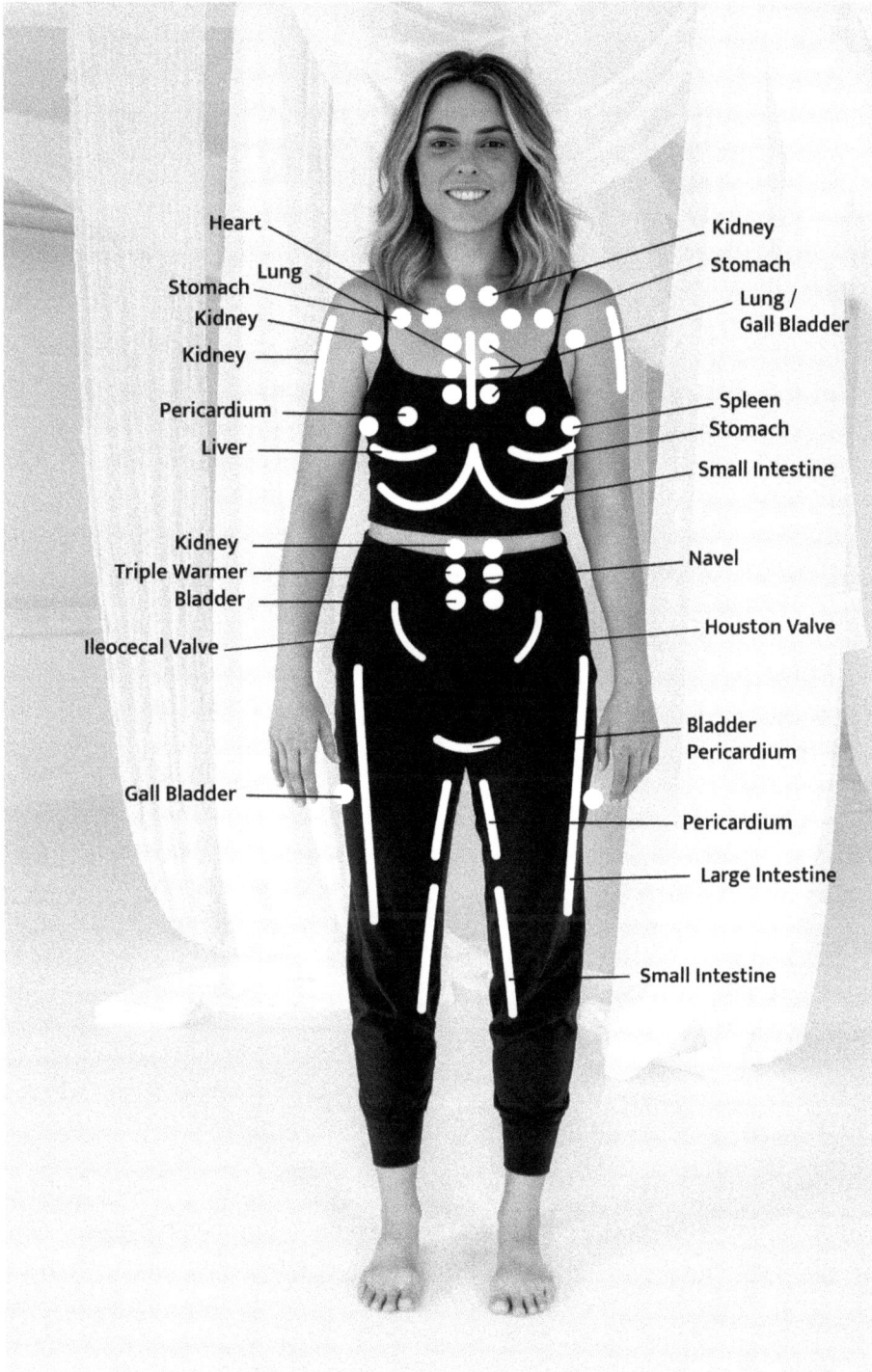

Heart
Lung
Stomach
Kidney
Kidney
Pericardium
Liver

Kidney
Stomach
Lung /
Gall Bladder
Spleen
Stomach
Small Intestine

Kidney
Triple Warmer
Bladder
Ileocecal Valve

Navel

Houston Valve

Bladder
Pericardium

Gall Bladder

Pericardium

Large Intestine

Small Intestine

Low Blood Counts

It's fairly common for cancer patients to have low platelet, white, or red blood counts or a combination thereof. Chemotherapy, surgery, radiation, and immunotherapy administered either independently or in combination can cause these conditions. The longer one is treated, the greater likelihood the effects will become cumulative. Bringing white blood levels back to within normal range can take months or even a year sometimes. The technical name for this condition is *neutropenia*. Neutropenia is a condition where a certain type of white cell that fights infection called *neutrophils* are low. Having neutropenia puts one at a greater risk of infection and contributes to fatigue. Working with the *xi cleft* points can help.

XI Cleft Points

Just as source points send energy to organs directly, xi cleft points have a specialized role to play. They are specific acupuncture points on meridian lines where blood, oxygen, and chi gather. Massaging, tapping, or holding these points circulates blood and chi throughout these meridians and the entire body.

When: This protocol should be done daily when first encountering low counts. It can be used for any blood-related issues.

Why: Working with xi clefts points is something one can easily do while sitting or lying down. They help support the blood and are also good to counteract pain, especially in the joints.

How: This can be done alone but, ideally, a partner would work on you.

1. Start with the yin points located on the interior of the legs. Work from the bottom of the leg up towards the knee.
2. Try to do both sides of the body at once. If you can't reach both legs or if it's too cumbersome, you can do one leg at a time.
3. Do the yin (inside) points first and then move to the yang (outside) points.
4. Even though these are specific acupuncture points, don't worry if you aren't exactly on the point. You can use two fingers and you will be close enough to the meridian to affect a change.

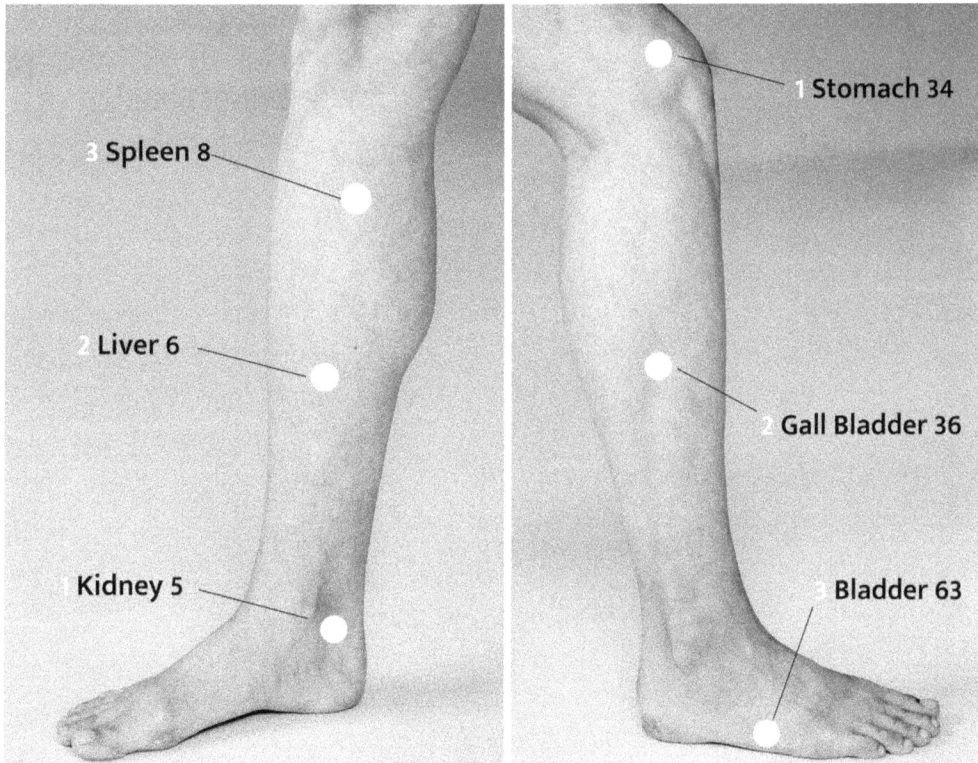

5. Start with the Kidney 5 point. Massage deeply to the count of five, making little circles on the point. It doesn't matter in which direction you move.

6. Keeping your fingers on the point, stop massaging and count to five.

7. Then, deeply massage the point again to the count of five and then stop to the count of five.

8. You will have created a pulsation at the point from this method. Do two more rounds of massaging and holding.

9. Repeat Steps 5 – 8 on the following points:

    Liver 6

    Spleen 8

10. You may find that some points are more tender than others. You can spend more time on these points as that indicates there is a blockage there.

11. Working from the knee towards the feet, repeat Steps 5 through 8 on the following points:

> Stomach 34
> Gall Bladder 36
> Bladder 63

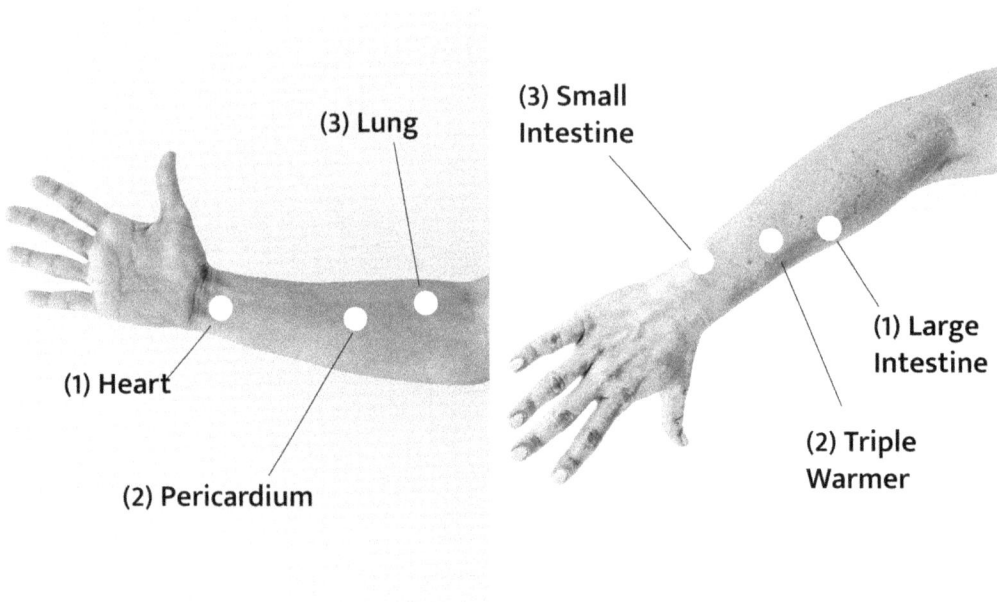

(3) Lung

(3) Small Intestine

(1) Heart

(2) Pericardium

(1) Large Intestine

(2) Triple Warmer

12. Move up to the arms, starting with the yin points on the inside of the arms. Start at the wrist points and move up the forearms. It will be difficult to massage both points simultaneously, so do one at a time or you could have someone do this for you.

13. Massage Heart 6 for five counts. Then rest for the count of five. Then do two more sets of five off, five on.

14. Repeat Steps 5-8 on the following points:

> Pericardium 4
> Lung 6
> Large Intestine 7
> Triple warmer 7
> Small intestine 6

15. Move to lung 6.

16. Turn your arm over and massage large intestine 7.

17. Move to triple warmer 7 and do the same procedure on this point.

18. End with small intestine 6.

19. Do this protocol daily.

Protecting Yourself Energetically

If you are immunocompromised due to your cancer treatment, there are things you can do to protect yourself energetically. I wrote earlier that our biofield is our first line of defense from environmental invaders. Doing the *Celtic Weave* (See Page107) and *Four Thumps* (See Page 152) exercises, will help to build your biofield and strengthen your thymus gland. Here are two more exercises that can help protect your biofield:

Zip and Hook Up

When: This should be done twice a day.

Why: The central and governing meridians function as an energetic spine and an anchor for our biofield. Tracing these in the direction in which they flow reinforces their connection, and holding anchor points along the meridian strengthens the biofield.

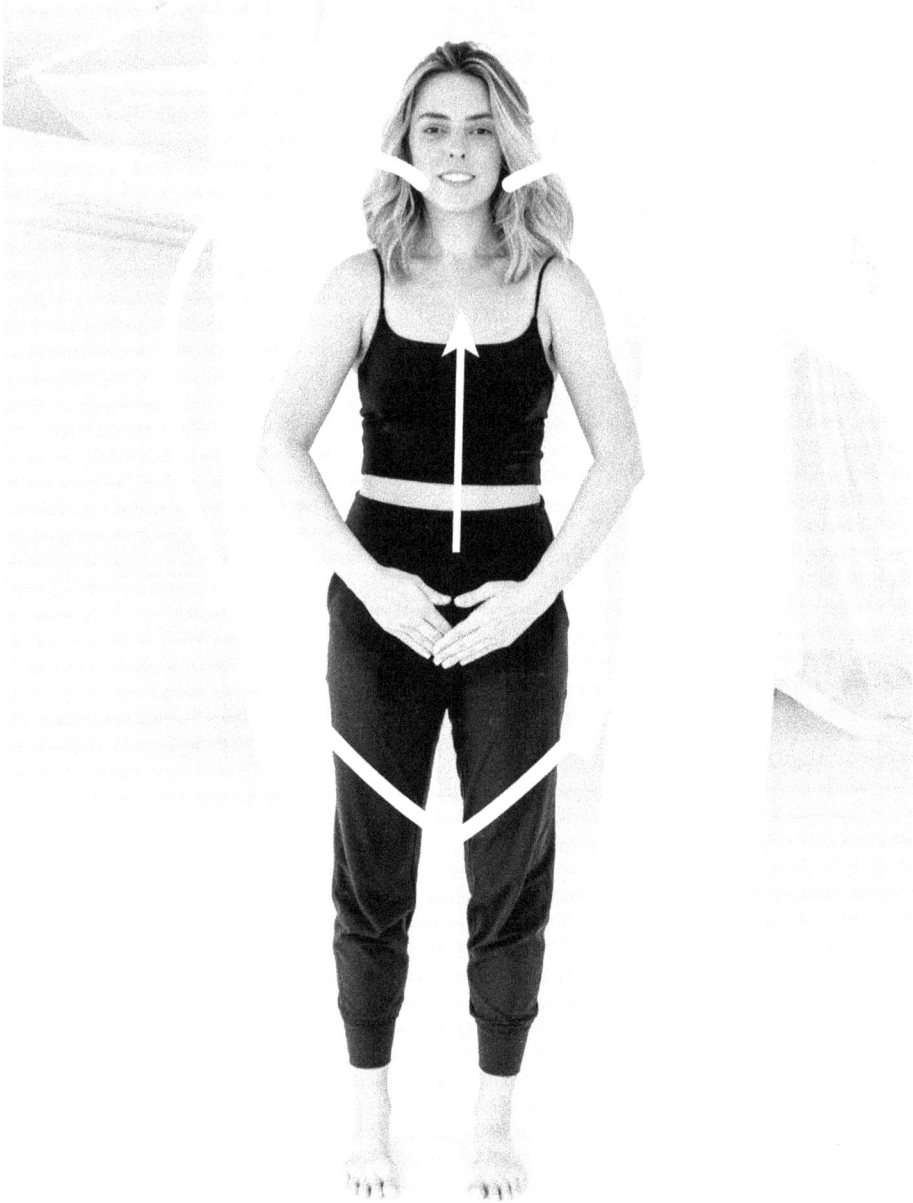

How:

1. Starting at your pubic bone, take your flat palm and draw a straight line up the center of your torso, extending your arms above your head and around your body.
2. Do this tracing three more times.
3. On the last pass, stop at your mouth and imagine there is a lock and key there. Turn the key to lock the point and throw it away.

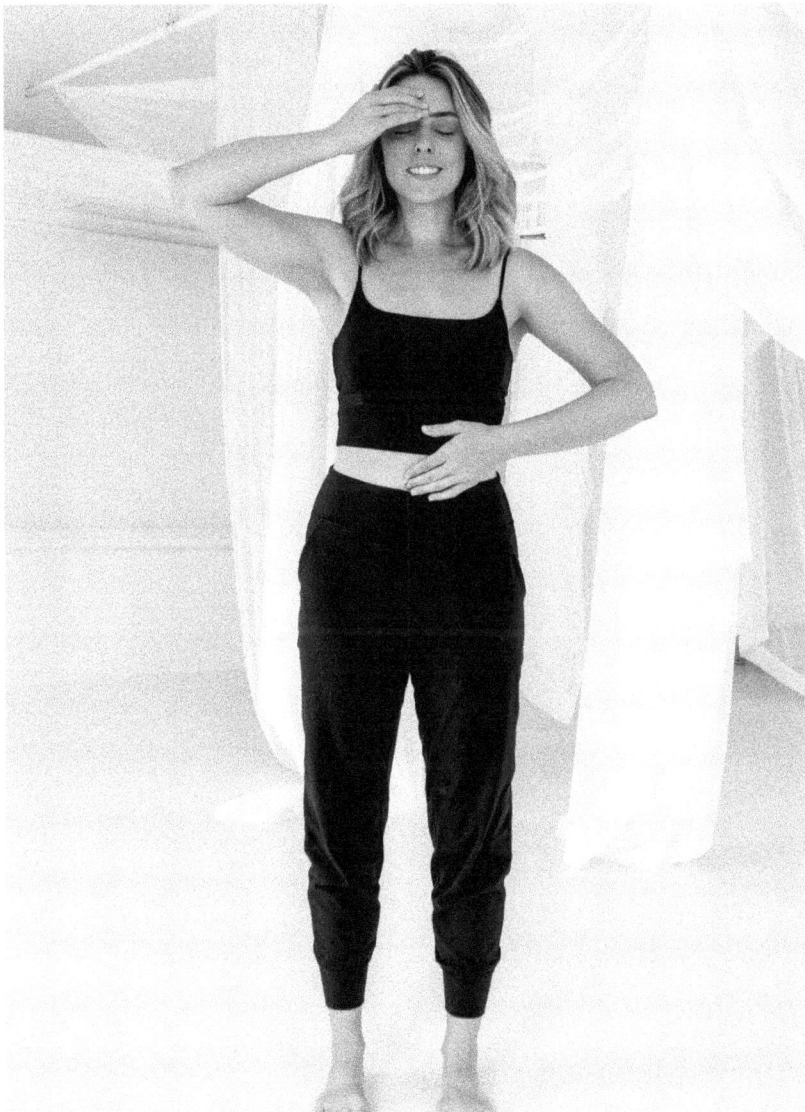

4. Now take your middle finger and place it in your navel.

5. Place your other middle finger either at your third eye or at the base of your neck.

6. Push in with your fingers and pull up on the points while you breathe in through your nose and exhale through your mouth.

7. Do this for at least 30 seconds to a minute.

Ideally, in our post-cancer experience, we're aiming to not just survive but to thrive. Recovery involves removing toxins, getting your energy back and staying positive. Each of these exercises can help you in that regard.

But what about the bigger questions facing you? You can approach your journey as narrowly or broadly as you choose to define it. Getting cancer was your body's way of getting your attention. Now that you're listening, what is it trying to tell you? Dr. David Pearlmutter, the famous neurologist and author, stated it this way, "The choices we make are what stops or starts the disease process in our bodies. The ball is in our court, not the doctors'. We are the arbiters of our health's destiny."[19] The paradigm of waiting for someone to "fix me" is a passive one. We have the power within ourselves to take responsibility for our health. Our lives may depend on it.

Final Thoughts

1. While undergoing treatment, have some kind of body work done if at all possible. This gives your body the clear and important message that not all touch is painful or intrusive. If you can't afford to pay someone, have a family member do it. (Of course, clear this with your medical team in case there is some contraindication.)

2. Build up your spiritual equity by having others pray for you or send you healing energy. Start a CaringBridge webpage so others can support you in your journey. Friends feel powerless and want to do something to help. This allows them to do something. All the encouragement I received helped me to stay strong and feel as though I could make it through. I looked forward to keeping friends and family up to date and getting their feedback.

3. Do as much self-care as possible: EEM, qigong, tai chi, or yoga—all of these will keep the life force energy moving in your body. Even if you are too sick to do them while you are undergoing treatment, do them as soon as possible after you are finished. Donna Eden has created something called the *Daily Energy Routine*, designed to support many of the energy systems in the body. The majority of these exercises are already detailed in this book, but there are others you can learn easily. If you do a YouTube search for *Eden Energy Medicine Daily Energy Routine*[18], you will find many demonstrations you can follow.

4. Move every day if possible. Exercise is critical to move toxins out of the body. Studies show that exercising even 150 minutes a week (30 minutes five times a week) can help prevent a cancer reoccurrence. The YMCA hosts the Livestrong Program for all cancer survivors, a free membership that includes classes and training for cancer patients and

their caregivers. I joined the program while I was in the middle of my treatment and I was so weak, I didn't think I could ever do classes or weights, but over time, I became stronger. If you can't use weights or machines, there are wonderful aqua classes that will get you moving in no time!

5. Move in nature. The healthiest place to exercise is in nature. We are designed to interact with nature and receive energetic elements from it. Donna Eden said once, "If we stay in nature long enough and live in harmony with it, our bodies can heal from anything."

6. Get your support team in place. As soon as you receive your diagnosis, begin to contact support or alternative practitioners. It can sometimes take weeks or months to get an appointment, so you want to move quickly. The most expensive practitioners are not necessarily the best.

7. Be your own best advocate. No one is going to advocate for you. YOU are the one in charge of you! If something doesn't feel right, ask questions. As much as possible, understand what is being done to your body. Do your own research. Even though doctors don't offer this information, there are often alternatives available to you that you might not know exist. Physicians are obligated to follow what is considered to be the "standard of care". If you choose not to do that or want some kind of different approach, medication or dosage, speak up. This lets them off the hook. As long as they document your chart, they must follow your wishes and they are legally protected. Don't wait until a problem arises that could develop into a late effect that never ends. For example, when I had symptoms of heart weakness, I stopped taking Herceptin until I knew the symptom was temporary.

8. Join Facebook cancer groups. There is a wealth of support and information on those pages; this is where you will meet your new tribe. One caveat: If you find you are being negatively affected by difficult or sad stories, take a break for awhile and don't come back until you are in a better frame of mind. These pages should be a source of education and inspiration, not fear and panic. They can be extremely helpful if you are struggling with something in particular and want to get feedback. Sometimes you don't have access to your medical team, or you want to hear directly from other patients: This is the best resource for that. I used them multiple times and found them to be invaluable. You can also share your story with others to support their journey.

9. Join cancer support groups. The same advice for the Facebook groups applies here. They can be a wonderful source of support, but they can also drag you down, so tread lightly.

10. Learn energy medicine! EEM and EFT can help you move out of survivor and into thriver status. We all want that. We don't want to be defined or limited by our cancer experience. I can honestly say I would not be anywhere near as resilient as I am post-cancer without either of these two modalities. They offer one of the easiest and fastest ways to get your triple warmer on board and not resist your treatment. Remember that energy medicine is like the weather. We can't see the air or how it moves the clouds, but we know that when it rains, the air has impacted our lives. It's the same with energy medicine: It's small, subtle changes that are made or maintained on a daily basis that make an impact. Combine different techniques; it will have a greater impact. If you can't do much, do what I call "Give a dog a bone approach." You might not be doing a tremendous amount of energy work, but if you do small things on a regular basis, like throwing a dog a bone, your triple warmer will work with you and trust you more. If you are lucky enough to live near an EEM practitioner, have them work on you on a regular basis or have them teach a loved one what they can do to help you on a daily basis. It can make a world of difference!

11. Look Inward: Every journey has a purpose and a destination. How did you find yourself here? What parts of your life facilitated this disease? In what ways were you being untrue to yourself or ignoring what your inner voice was trying to tell you? What did you put off in your life, waiting for "later"? Now that "later" is here, what are you going to do about it? What if doing it might make the difference between life or death?

12. A note to caregivers and loved ones: Unfortunately, you are on this journey, too. Caregivers are often the ones that pay the price because everyone is focused on the patient, and no one takes care of the caregiver. All of the self-care exercises explained here can and should be done by you as well. Remember, you are not the healer; you are not responsible for what happens to your loved one. You are merely the catalyst or facilitator for your loved one's body to balance itself.

Kimberly shares these insights with you:

Caregivers, you need to take care of yourself. You cannot show up for your loved one without a full cup of your own. This is powerful stuff we're clearing and working with. We are warriors walking alongside our people, brandishing powerful medicine. We need to keep our armor intact, our bodies grounded, our spirits aligned, and our vibration high. If you cannot do it for yourself, do it for the person you love. Take yourself on a journey during this experience of how to love yourself enough to take care of this life, body, and the time here you were given.

Postscript

January 19, 2023

I am in the middle of drafting this book and reliving my experience as I write it. It has been emotionally painful to write this book because I had forgotten many parts of my journey and compiling it has forced me to retrace those steps.

I will be having my port removed tomorrow. The port I initially viewed as a failure has become a friend. I've even given it a name: Portman. Portman has been with me through thick and thin. He helped me get through my infusions with less pain. He's become a crutch on which I could rely. There is a certain amount of trepidation at the thought of letting him go. Having him gone means all future blood draws will be directly on my arm, a process I dislike. But more than that, having him removed is a clear indicator that this trip is over. I wanted to at least give him a burial ceremony to thank him for his service, but alas, Nurse Nathalie says they most likely will not let me have him.

As much as I have been critical of the traditional medical model through this journey, I feel as though I have made my peace with Western medicine. It certainly has its shortcomings, but thanks to research and technology, it is keeping people alive longer. Is it perfect? No, not at all. In a perfect world, it would work hand in glove with alternative modalities such as energy medicine and naturopathy. I was one of the lucky ones who could incorporate multiple modalities to support, protect, and assist my body through my cancer treatment. If this book helps you to do the same, my efforts will not have been in vain.

Acknowledgements

There are so many people without whose support, I could not have written this book. First, I want to thank my husband, Jean-Pierre, who drove me to countless appointments, accompanied me to my chemo infusions and was my Number 1 cheerleader throughout this project. Next, my daughters, Kimberly Baer and Nathalie Howell and their husbands, Danny and Zach who housed, nurtured and nursed me during my most difficult and painful periods. To my son, Jonathan, whose positive attitude and perseverance during his cancer journey were an inspiration to me. Then, all of my family, friends, colleagues, students and clients who sent me healing energy, prayers and love throughout my ordeal, in particular, Sylvia Sturm and the Smith Center for Healing and the Arts in Washington, DC. Their volunteers sent me Reiki energy every Thursday afternoon for more than a year! To Anna and Mehrdad Mizani, who have demonstrated throughout my life what true friendship means. To Donna Eden and David Feinstein, who provided loving energetic support during this time. A special thank you to the doctors and medical staff at all of the hospitals in DC and Boston; without their expertise and care I would not be here today. Thank you to my editors, Louise Strait and Joelle Hann and my readers, Nancy Brown, Linda Geronilla, Kimberly, Nathalie and Jean-Pierre. I am grateful to my book designer, Jonathan Gullery, who helped me move this project to completion. A shout out to Casey Haley of Joppa Photography and Kim who modeled the energy medicine poses beautifully. And finally, my healers, Tom Tam, Peggy Moseley, Heather Gary and Kimberly, without whose healing touch, my journey would not have been so smooth.

Endnotes

1. See, e.g., *The Science of Subtle Energy: The Healing Power of Dark Matter*, by Yury Kron, Park Street Press, 2022; *Energy Medicine, The Scientific Basis*, by James Oschman, Churchill Livingston Press, 2000.

2. *Energy Medicine: Balance Your Body's Energies for Optimum Health, Joy, and Vitality*, by Donna Eden, Paragon Press, 1999.

3. See, e.g., *The EFT Manual*, by Gary Craig, Energy Psychology Press, 2008; *The Tapping Manual: The Complete Guide to Using EFT (Emotional Freedom Techniques) for Common Issues,* by Dawson Church, PhD., Energy Psychology Press, 2018.

4. The many modalities I used during treatment:

   Acupuncture
   Active Release Therapy
   Alkaline diet
   Calcium Bentonite Clay
   Chris Wark's Anti-cancer diet
   Cranial Sacral Therapy
   Emotion Code
   Eden Energy Medicine
   Energy Psychology (EFT)
   Epsom salt and baking soda baths
   Essential Oils
   Fenbendazole
   Good-Bye Lupus Diet
   Homeopathy

Intermittent Fasting

Jin Shin Jitsu

Livestrong Program - Local YMCA

Matcha Tea

Naturopathy

Oil Pulling

Parts Work

Quantum Healing

Qigong

Reiki

Remote Healing

Somatic Experiencing

Supplements

Tuina Massage

THC/CBD

Tong Ren Healing

Vitamin C – High Dose

Yoga

5. *Personal Writings,* by Albert Camus, Random House Press, 1957.

6. See, e.g., *No Bad Parts, Healing Trauma and Restoring Wholeness with the Internal Family Systems Model,* by Richard C. Schwartz, PhD., Sounds True, 2021; *Internal Family Systems Therapy, Second Edition,* by Richard C. Schwartz and Martha Sweezy, Guilford Press, 2019. *Imagery In You: Mining For Treasure In Your Inner World*, by Jenny Garrison, Outskirts Press, 2006.

7. Tom Tam has written more than thirty books about the relationship between bioelectricity in the body and illness, with a particular emphasis on cancer. Here is the link for Tong Ren Station: www.tongrenstation.com.

8. See, e.g., https://www.youtube.com/watch?v=Ac08kMK-dyI&ab_channel=TylerTrahan; https://www.youtube.com/watch?v=YpG7xCkiq0A&ab_channel=HackMotivation.

9. Caring Bridge Webpage Setup*: https://www.caringbridge.org/how-it-works?&msclkid=1e-77f9a19e9c18efa1cd9cc9054bb639&gclsrc=3p.ds.*

10. All PubMed studies referenced can be found at: www.pubmed.gov.

11. *Goodbye Lupus: How a Medical Doctor Healed Herself Naturally With Supermarket Foods,* Dr. Brooke Goldner, 2015.

12. Lymphatic Education and Research Network's Patient Symposium 2019, Chuck Ehlich, MS, MBA. https://www.youtube.com/watch?v=krBvYTfxJks&ab_channel=LymphaticEducation%26ResearchNetwork%28LE%26RN%29.

13. *Trastuzumab Emtansine for Residual Invasive HER2-Positive Breast Cancer,* New England Journal of Medicine, February 14, 2001.

14. Active Release Technique: www.activerelease.com.

15. Livestrong Program at the YMCA: https://www.ymca.org/what-we-do/healthy-living/fitness/livestrong.

16. *Pioneering an Integrative Nursing Practice in a Boston Cancer Institution,* presented at the 2nd International Integrative Nursing Society Conference Study by Eileen Valentini, RN, Dana Farber Hospital, Boston, MA, 2017.

17. Science Daily, *Touch therapy helps reduce pain, nausea in cancer patients,* University of Kentucky, Markey Cancer Center, June 26, 2012.

18. *Power Up Your Brain: The Neuroscience of Enlightenment,* by David Permutter, FACN and Alberto Villoldo, PhD. Hay House, 2011.

19. Donna Eden's Daily Energy Routine: Youtube: *https://www.youtube.com/watch?v=Di5Ua44iuXc&ab_channel=DonnaEdenEnergyMedicine.*

Glossary

Aura or Biofield: The biofield has historically been called the aura, the field, the subtle body or, in Hindu traditions, the Nadis. Donna Eden explains it well in her book *Energy Medicine*: "The aura is like our body's spacesuit. It protects us but it also functions like a radio antenna; it also attracts energy to us." Another appropriate analogy is that of the earth and it's atmosphere. Although it can't be seen, the atmosphere protects the earth. If a hole develops in the atmosphere, that event can have detrimental consequences. It's the same with the human biofield. If it has holes or tears in it, the physical body won't be protected and consequently, one's health can be negatively impacted. The biofield should extend about an arm's length in every direction from the body: around, above and below. The space contained within that space should have lots and lots of crossover patterns. The more crossover patterns it has, the healthier the body will be. Within the biofield sit the chakras.

Celtic Weave: One of the nine energy systems, the celtic weave contains all of the other eight energy systems within it. It networks through and around the body in small and large figure 8 patterns. Donna Eden calls it the 'connective tissue' of the energy body. The biofield, chakras and tibetan rings all sit within it.

Chakras: Chakra is a Sanskrit word that means "disc" and refers to energy centers that are located along the spine. There are seven main chakras: root, womb, solar plexus, heart, throat, third eye and crown. Each chakra has seven layers. Chakras exchange energy with the biofield and send energy into the body by means of the endocrine system. Every organ that resides within the space of a chakra is impacted by that chakra. Yogis use yoga and pranayama (breath work) to control or shift the energy of the chakra system. Each chakra also has a color associated with it: Root-red, womb-orange, solar plexus-yellow, heart-green, throat-light blue, third eye-blue, crown-indigo or in some traditions, white. Each chakra also represents a period of time in one's life and all memories are imprinted within the chakra. There are emotions or themes associated with each chakra as well: Root-survival, womb-creativity, solar plexus-identity and power, heart-love and healing, throat-communication, third eye-awareness, crown-spirituality. The Eden Method teaches that you can clear and strengthen each of these chakras in order to balance both the energy system itself and the organs that correspond to a particular chakra.

Chi: The life force that flows and sustains our bodies. Many ancient healing traditions work with this energy and call it by different names: prana, qi, chi, spirit etc. (The terms energy and chi are used interchangeably in this book.)

Electrics: This system is the densest of the nine energy systems and consequently, can be measured by medical instruments. EKGs and EEGs are examples of how science maps this energy system. Science also understands that our bones produce piezoelectricity every time we move. Every cell in our body has a positive and negative charge and these polarities can be reversed in illness or if there is a lack of oxygen in the body. Donna Eden describes the electrical system as intimately permeating all the other energy systems of the body in the same way that liquid is part of an organ but not the organ itself. She teaches that balancing the electrical system is critical for cancer patients. In 1955, Dr. Otto Warburg discovered that cancer cells use an anaerobic process of respiration to produce energy. Anaerobic means "without oxygen." Warburg found that you can reverse this process simply by adding oxygen – but only if you do it early enough to cancer cells. Low oxygenation accelerates malignant progression and metastasis, thereby creating a poorer prognosis irrespective of which cancer treatment is used. This could explain why cancer patients who exercise up to 150 minutes per week have a significantly lower risk of relapse. Many alternative cancer specialists understand that a lack of oxygenation can cause cancer cells to reproduce. A lack of oxygenation can also reverse polarity within the cells so working with the electrics is important in cancer treatment. An electric protoco should be performed by an EEM practitioner, therefore it is not contained in this book.

Emotional Freedom Technique (EFT): EFT is a healing method that addresses negative emotions, pain or trauma and affects change by tapping acupressure points while focusing on the negative emotion, pain or trauma. There are multiple techniques within the skill set that can adapt and adjust to an individual's needs so that whatever the issue is, an effective response to that issue can be elicited. EFT is derived from various theories of alternative medicine including acupuncture, Neuro-linguistic programming, energy medicine, and Thought Field Therapy. There are scores of studies demonstrating its effectiveness.

Energy Testing: A biofeedback mechanism that conveys information from the body to reveal what is out of balance or in need of support. It also assesses the flow of energy through a muscle. Each muscle in the body is associated with a meridian. Muscle testing assesses the strength of a muscle but energy testing assesses the energy of a meridian that flows through a muscle that is governed by a particular meridian. By utilizing this technique, it allows information that cannot be perceived with the five senses to be revealed to the client and practitioner. Energy testing is used only to gain information about the body being tested and how to bring that body into balance. Techniques to get baseline testing include using true or false statements and weakening a muscle associated with a meridian and then strengthening it. It can be used to convey information about the body and to test substances to see whether they are compatible with and will be metabolized well.

Five Elements: TCM teaches that nature is comprised of five elements: water, wood, fire, earth and metal. Since the human body is part of nature, it is composed of these same five elements. Each organ is associated with one of these elements and there is a relationship between these elements within the body. Donna Eden calls these the "five rhythms" because, like music, they ebb and flow in the body and how they interact with one another can have a positive or negative impact on one's health.

Gaits: These are the spaces that exist between the bones of the hands (phalanges) and feet (metatarsals). Massaging these places can help move stuck energy out of the body through the tips of the fingers and toes, each of which is the beginning or endpoint of a meridian.

Grid: Donna Eden describes the basic grid as the "bones" of the energy body. Just as the bones support the muscles, tissues and other structures of the physical body, the grid is the energetic infrastructure of the other eight energy systems. There are eight major grids and 58 minor grids. There are four major grids on the front of the body and four on the back. A break in a major grid can have a negative and long-term impact on the health of that body. Illness, trauma, or an accident can break a grid and it does not usually repair itself spontaneously. The best analogy is to think of it like a car's chassis; if the chassis is damaged in some way, the car can be driven, but the driver must continually compensate for the damage. Healing a broken grid is the deepest of all energy work and can have a positive and profound impact on one's life and health.

Homolateral Energies: Homolateral energies occur when the left and right hemispheres of the brain are not operating or communicating in an optimal manner. Babies are born with homolateral energies, but as they begin to crawl, the neural connections between the hemispheres begin to form via the corpus callosum. Under stress, however, the body can revert to this homolateral energetic neurological state which has negative implications for both the mind and the body.

Meridians: Meridians are energy pathways that feed, govern and energize the body's organs and physiology. Each meridian contains hundreds of tiny, distinct reservoirs of heat and electro-magnetic energy called acupuncture or acupressure points that can be stimulated with needles or pressure to release or balance blocked energy in the meridian channel. Their network is as extensive as the circulatory and lymph systems. TCM mapped these energy flows thousands of years ago and science is starting to be able to map them as well. Manipulating these energetic pathways in order to heal or balance a body is at the core of TCM. There is actually just one long meridian. Central and Governing are two meridians that are not bilateral and operate independently of an organ. The other twelve are bilateral and pass through the organs for which they are named: spleen, heart, small intestine, bladder, kidney, pericardium, triple warmer, gall bladder, liver, lung, large intestine and stomach.

Neurolymphatic Points: First discovered by Dr. Frank Chapman, an osteopath, in the 1920s.

These points are located on the front and back of the body and correspond to each organ and meridian. Connected to the meridians via the radiant circuits, they are reflex points that turn on and activate the lymphatic aspect of the corresponding meridian or organ. Massaging them deeply not only turns on the lymphatic system with respect to that organ, it also balances both the physical and emotional aspect of that organ and meridian.

Neurovascular Points: These are acupuncture points that are found primarily on the head. They deal specifically with emotional or mental stress, but working with them can also positively affect the physical body since many physical issues have an emotional component. Holding these points lightly brings blood, oxygen and chi back to the head and helps counter stress response in the nervous system.

Radiant Circuits: Known as "extraordinary vessels" or "strange flows" in TCM, these energy channels predate meridians. They are the life force that exists within all living organisms. Unlike meridians, they don't move in fixed patterns so, if activated, they can go anywhere in the body that needs healing. Activating these channels fortifies the meridians as well as bodily system functions such as hormone distribution, circulation and so forth. If they are dormant, it can be more difficult for the body to heal from surgery or an illness and one might have less vitality.

Scrambled Energy: Similar to homolateral energies, scrambled energies involve a breakdown in communication between the right and left hemispheres of the brain as well as an energetic disconnection between the prefrontal cortex and limbic system of the brain. A sense of confusion, muddled thinking and overwhelm are the hallmark signs of this condition.

Shock Points: When there is a shock to the body, it enters through the feet. It then reverberates throughout the body while the triple warmer system tries to process it. Holding specific points on the foot with pressure can help release stored shock in the body thereby helping the body heal from the trauma.

Source Points: These are acupuncture points that are akin to "holding tanks" for energy. They contain more energy than other acupuncture points and they directly feed the organ for which they are named. Massaging, tapping or holding them can help revitalize an otherwise compromised meridian or organ.

Substance Repatterning: A technique that assists the mind, body and nervous system to acclimate to a particular substance, medication or supplement. By working with acupuncture points, it retrains the body to not resist and come into harmony with the substance.

Tibetan Rings: Contained within the celtic weave energy system, these figure eight patterns have been called tibetan rings because they are part of that nation's ancient healing practice. They are large and small figure 8 shapes that follow the body's anatomy. They function like energetic fascia for the body parts they contain. Working with these can help strengthen the immune system, counteract pain and facilitate healing from surgery or illness.

Triple Warmer: Triple warmer is both a meridian and a radiant circuit. It has multiple jobs in the body and is not tied to a particular organ. It is known as "triple burner" or "triple heater" in TCM because it is comprised of lower, middle and upper "burner'" that coordinate the organs and their bodily functions within each region. Along with spleen meridian, it governs the immune system. When it functions as a meridian, it performs it's physiological aspects. When acting as a radiant circuit, it operates on a broader level and governs not just the immune system, but also the body's stress response. This aspect is of paramount importance because when the body is in stress response, all other systems of the body: respiration, circulation, reproduction, digestive and immune response will be sublimated and negatively impacted. If the body stays in stress response long enough, significant and potentially deadly consequences may ensue. Any illness in the body is caused by an imbalance between triple warmer and spleen meridians in addition to whatever organ is involved. Learning how to balance these two meridians is imperative to heal) the body of any disease.

Triple Warmer Reactivity: Triple warmer reactivity occurs when a person has been in fight, flight or freeze stress response for so long that the body does not know how to come back to a healthy or balanced response. It becomes stuck in the heightened stress response and consequently responds to all stimuli as a stressor. Living in this state can have profoundly negative implications at the mental, emotional and physical level. The closest analogy in traditional medicine is post-traumatic stress disorder.

Xi Cleft Points: Xi cleft points are acupuncture points that help circulate blood, oxygen and chi throughout the body. They sit on points where the blood vessels and meridians meet. Massaging these deeply can help facilitate a smoother flow of chi, blood and oxygen thereby assisting the healing process.

About the Author

Dianne Faure was an attorney at the U.S. Civil Rights Commission, who specialized in health discrimination. Her own health deteriorated over time, preventing her from working. However, her encounter with Eden Energy Medicine proved to be life-changing. She was so impressed by its effectiveness that she studied with Donna Eden for five years, becoming an Advanced Eden Energy Practitioner and Fundamentals Teacher. After successfully healing herself of her chronic autoimmune issues, Dianne realized that Energy Medicine was her true passion. She became a Licensed Massage Therapist and opened a private practice in Bethesda, MD. In addition, Dianne was on the Medical Staff at the Casey Health Institute, where she taught physicians, chiropractors, acupuncturists, clinical psychologists, naturopaths, nutritionists, and patients the benefits of Energy Medicine. She also taught at the Johns Hopkins Kimmel Cancer Center in Baltimore, MD.

Dianne has been certified as an Energy Psychologist and Coach through EFT Universe and has also been trained in Somatic Experiencing, Celtic Shamanism, and Star Magic Healing. She has been interviewed on the Gaia Network's *Dr. Sue Morter Show*, on the *Curiosity and Consciousness* podcast, and has been a presenter at two *Energy Fest* Conferences. Having overcome cancer, Dianne has resumed her career as a teacher, coach and Energy Medicine Practitioner.

Index

www.ingramcontent.com/pod-product-compliance
Lightning Source LLC
Chambersburg PA
CBHW042338030426
42335CB00030B/3389